QUICK GUIDES

Evening
Primrose Oil

LIZ EARLE'S
QUICK GUIDES

Evening Primrose Oil

B◈XTREE

First published in Great Britain in 1994 by Boxtree Limited,
Broadwall House, 21 Broadwall, London SE1 9PL

The right of Liz Earle to be identified as Author of this Work has
been asserted by her in accordance with the Copyright, Designs and
Patents Act 1988

10 9 8 7 6 5 4 3 2 1

ISBN: 0 7522 1619 8

Text design by Blackjacks
Cover design by Hammond Hammond

Printed and bound in Great Britain by
Mackays of Chatham PLC, Chatham, Kent

A CIP catalogue entry for this book is available from
the British Library

Contents

ACKNOWLEDGEMENTS

I am grateful to Sarah Hamilton Fleming for helping to produce this book. Also to the many research institutes and manufacturers who have so generously provided copies of clinical papers and details of the many medical trials using evening primrose oil. I am also indebted to the talented team at Boxtree, my agent Rosemary Sandberg and Claire Bowles Publicity for their unfailing enthusiasm and support.

Introduction

Evening primrose oil is one of my favourite supplements as it has quite literally saved my skin. As someone with eczema I have first-hand experience of the very real benefits of this miraculous oil. Since I began taking it almost a decade ago, my skin has never looked or felt better. But there is so much more to this humble plant than the powers of skin rejuvenation. This *Quick Guide* reveals how it can help an incredibly wide range of ailments, from PMS to symptoms of the menopause, to diabetes, arthritis and even hyperactivity in children. And while it is by no means a cure-all, it does offer some surprising advantages for those who try it. So if you are one of the many millions who take their daily capsules, or if you simply want to find out whether the oil might help your own health, read on to discover the magic of the evening primrose.

Liz Earle

— 1 —
The Plant and Its History

Oil of evening primrose is Britain's biggest selling supplement for women and there has been extensive research into its many hidden powers. The oil comes from the seeds of the evening primrose; the plant is not at all like a common primrose but is tall and spiky with vivid, egg-yolk yellow flowers. It only blooms in the evening (hence its name) and thrives on poor soil and extreme weather conditions.

The evening primrose can be traced back 70,000 years to Central America and Mexico where the North American Indian medicine men were the first to make use of its extraordinary healing powers. They made poultices from its leaves to sooth aches and sprains and used the juice from its roots as a cough mixture. They also brewed up the plant's seed pods to make anti-inflammatory infusions. It is the seed pods that contain the secret of the evening primrose plant's more recent success. These seeds are rich in oil which is a rare source of the essential fatty acid GLA (gamma-linolenic acid). Essential fatty acids (EFAs) are needed by the skin to maintain its tone and elasticity as well as having other important biochemical effects, but gamma-linolenic acid does much more, as will be explained in this *Quick Guide*.

Evening primrose spread from America throughout the world. Botanists first brought it to Europe from Virginia in 1614 in order to study it. In 1650, the English herbalist Nicholas Culpeper recorded his use of the evening primrose, saying 'it opens obstructions of the liver and spleen, provokes urine, is good for the dropsy if infused in common drink.' (Dropsy is the old-fashioned word for oedema, or swelling, and it is not a disease in itself but a sign of kidney or heart disease.) However, most of the strains of evening primrose which we have in Britain arrived accidentally during the next century on cargo ships carrying cotton. As cotton is very light, extra soil was used as ballast. The soil, containing stray seeds of evening primrose, was dumped on reaching port. Evening primrose began to spring up in areas surrounding ports such as Liverpool and, even today, the descendants of these plants can be found near such ports.

In Europe, the evening primrose became known as 'King's Cure All' by those who were aware of its marvellous medicinal properties. Despite this, the evening primrose has been virtually ignored for centuries, with only a few herbalists showing any interest in it. Old herbals describe the evening primrose plant as being astringent and sedative, and its oil as being helpful in treating gastro-intestinal disorders, whooping cough, asthma, female complaints and wound healing. It is only fairly recently, though, that evening primrose oil has gained a high profile. In 1917 a German scientist called Unger examined the plant and discovered that the seeds contained 15 percent oil, which could be extracted using light petroleum. Medical attention was then focused solely on the oil-bearing seeds of this remarkable plant. This oil was originally analysed in 1919 by Heiduschka and Luft, who discovered and identified GLA (gamma-linolenic acid) and other essential fatty acids for the first time. Later, in 1927, three German scientists repeated the Heiduschka and Luft test and made a more detailed analysis of the chemical structure of GLA.

Twenty-two years later Dr J.P. Riley, a British biochemist in the Department of Industrial Chemistry at Liverpool University, decided to analyse the evening primrose oil himself using modern techniques. He was excited when he also found this unique gamma-linolenic acid, but it was not until the 1960s that British scientists began to examine the oil's health-giving properties.

The history of the evening primrose is like a tale of 'rags to riches'. Not so long ago the evening primrose was looked upon as a humble weed found along waysides, but now many farmers, in their efforts to diversify, grow evening primrose as a commercial crop. The manufacturing of evening primrose oil has become big business.

From Flower to Capsule

Harvesting evening primrose oil is by no means a simple process. To start with, there are over 1,600 types of evening primrose and each has different characteristics. The different strains are collected together from around the world for the breeding programme. Pollen from the 'parent' plant is used to fertilise the female plant. Each season the different plants' characteristics are examined and the best plants are used to establish the next generations. It takes about fifteen years of cross-pollination to produce a new variety and in this time 99 percent of the plants would have been discarded. The seeds from the chosen variety are sent to farmers in up to fifteen different countries to grow on to provide seeds for oil. Two kilograms of seeds are yielded per hectare of land. The seeds are sown in August and harvested by machine the following October.

Once the seeds have been harvested, they are then sieved. Alien seeds are separated; air blowers eliminate lighter seeds and the heavier ones are shaken out. The good seed is then stored until required. Oil is extracted using a series of rollers which crack the seed cases, exposing the oil cells. The seeds are then soaked in a solvent which absorbs the oil, making a solution called micella. Then, through a process of distillation, the solvent is removed leaving behind the pure evening primrose oil. This is then instantly sealed in air-tight polythene-lined drums because air contact corrupts the purity of the oil and can turn it rancid. Finally, the oil is taken from the drum and injected between two strips of soft gelatine. At this stage vitamin E (also renowned for its cell-regenerating properties) is commonly added. This vitamin is essential for the body to make full use of the beneficial properties of the oil. So, when choosing a supplement, look for one with added vitamin E. The laborious process of extracting evening primrose oil, and the fact that it takes around 2,000 tiny seeds to fill a single capsule of oil does make the final product expensive.

The Medical Evidence

The first medical experiments on evening primrose oil in Britain took place during the 1960s. These were carried out on rats who were given a diet lacking in essential fatty acids. After a couple of weeks they experienced loss of hair and skin problems. They were then divided into two groups; one was fed on linoleic acid (an essential fatty acid found in polyunsaturated vegetable oils) and the other group was fed gamma-linolenic acid (found in evening primrose oil). The results were astounding: the rats who had been given GLA recovered more rapidly than the other group and evidence revealed that the GLA was far more effectively used by the cells of all the important tissues and organs of the body than the linoleic acid. Much of the research during the 1960s was carried out by John Williams and his company, Bio-Oil Research. He was the first British biochemist to take a real interest in evening primrose and, as a result of his work, there has been a great deal of further research into the oil.

The success of these early experiments encouraged biochemists and other scientists to begin many more research projects. The next test was an investigation of the effect of the GLA in regulating blood cholesterol production in a group of rabbits being fed a diet high in animal fats and to compare the results with a group of rabbits fed a normal diet. The results showed that the GLA in evening primrose oil could control blood cholesterol levels. More research followed revealing other possible uses of evening primrose oil. One important study discovered that evening primrose oil could be beneficial in the treatment of multiple sclerosis (MS). A leading specialist in MS, Professor E.J. Field, who was at Newcastle University in 1974, discovered that evening primrose oil can be effective in reducing the severity and frequency of relapses in MS patients. Many people suffering from the disease now take evening primrose oil capsules on his advice.

ESSENTIAL FATTY ACIDS

Another enterprising doctor, David Horrobin, who was also at Newcastle in the 1970s, became interested in the oil as a result of his work on schizophrenia and prostaglandins (hormone-like compounds which regulate many bodily functions) and their precursors, the essential fatty acids (EFAs), found in foods. EFAs have many uses: they provide energy, maintain body temperature, insulate the nerves and cushion and protect body tissues. EFAs are found in polyunsaturated foods such as sunflower, safflower and olive oils, fish oils and many more oils found in nuts and seeds.

It is important to distinguish between trans-fatty acids and essential fatty acids. Fatty acids vary in structure and may be saturated or unsaturated. In chemical terms, if the carbon chains contain the maximum number of hydrogen atoms, the acids are said to be saturated, while those that lack a certain number of hydrogen atoms are said to be unsaturated.

Saturated fats are mostly of animal origin such as red meat and dairy products and we should avoid them because they interfere with the beneficial activity of essential fatty acids. Saturated fats make up between 85 percent and 93 percent of all fatty acids contained in Western diets. Processed vegetable oils, which make up over 90 percent of all oil available in the shops, are like saturated fats and they contain trans-fatty acids which interfere with the enzyme which changes the linoleic acid found in polyunsaturated foods into GLA. Sunflower, safflower, walnut, grapeseed, soya bean and rapeseed oil all contain essential fatty acids.

It is only in the last few years that the very important role that essential fatty acids (EFAs) play in the body has been investigated and at last acknowledged. Not so long ago doctors would never have thought to ask people what food they ate when treating them. When people suffered from a condition they went to the doctor to be prescribed drugs, when more often than not, their illness could probably have been helped or even cured simply by changing their diet. Many neurological diseases cannot be cured by drugs, but recent research has shown that the condition of some patients can be massively improved by a change in diet and taking supplements of certain essential fatty acids.

This major development in biochemistry has only very recently filtered through to the media, with even Hollywood acknowledging it in the film *Lorenzo's Oil*, based on a true story. Nick Nolte and Susan Sarandon act out the roles of the real-life couple whose son, Lorenzo, suffers from an incurable and devastating disease known as Adrenoleukodystrophy (ALD). This rare disease is passed from the mother only to male offspring. The symptoms start with the child behaving abnormally and throwing temper tantrums. The disease goes on to destroy the person's brain, making him deaf, dumb and blind and eventually, usually around two years after diagnosis, he dies. Because the disease affected so few children in America, no funding had been put forward to search for a cure and very little was known about it. This was until the early 1980s, when Lorenzo Odone developed ALD and his parents were determined to find a cure. His father spent every spare second of the day reading obscure papers on biochemistry until he knew almost as much as the doctors. Through this couple's determination to cure their son, all the experts on ALD from around the world were brought together and a cure was finally discovered in the form of oleic and erucic acid. From examining Lorenzo's blood it was discovered that it contained an abnormally high level of saturated fat. This had built up and was destroying the myelin sheath which protects the nerve fibres in the brain. When Lorenzo was given oleic acid in the form of monounsaturated olive oil, the amount of saturated fat in his blood dropped by 50 percent. However, oleic acid was not high up enough in the chain of essential fatty acids to stop the development of the disease. Erucic acid from rapeseed oil was then tested. Soon after Lorenzo was given a mixture of oleic and erucic acid, his blood levels returned to normal, and although he was on the verge of death, his condition began to improve. Before this treatment Lorenzo was unable to talk, swallow, move or even breathe without the aid of a machine and now he can move and can even articulate sounds. Since the discovery of the power of essential fatty acids in the 1980s and thanks to the determination of the Odone family, hundreds of children with ALD can now lead more normal lives.

To emphasise the importance of essential fatty acids, the World Health Organization advises that essential fatty acids should make up at least 3 percent of our total calorific intake and this should be increased to 5–6 percent for children and breast-feeding women.

During his research, the British chemist Dr David Horrobin discovered that many seemingly unrelated conditions such as atopic eczema, pre-menstrual syndrome, diabetes and ageing all involve the body being unable to use linoleic acid correctly. In each case, the problem was found to be caused by the body's inability to convert linoleic acid to gamma-linolenic acid (GLA). The next step was to find a source of GLA which could correct this deficiency. His work found that evening primrose oil is a particularly good source of GLA, and the gamma-linolenic acid found in evening primrose oil is biologically important as it affects much of the enzyme activity in our body. Every process that takes place within us is triggered by the action of various enzymes, including the production of prostaglandins.

PROSTAGLANDINS

Prostaglandins are hormone-like substances that regulate bodily functions including blood pressure, digestion and inflammation. Since the discovery in the 1930s, by the Swedish scientist U.S. von Euler, of a substance in the prostate gland which he named prostaglandin, approximately thirty-six different prostaglandins have been identified – they occur in every cell in the body.

The study of prostaglandins, still in its early stages, is another fascinating field in fat and oil biochemistry. Prostaglandins regulate the movement of material between individual cells, control cell-to-cell communication and the transmission of signals between nerve cells. Although biochemists have yet to pin-point exactly how all prostaglandins work at a molecular level, these hormone-like substances seem to exercise control over just about anything and everything in the body.

Unlike hormones, prostaglandins are not secreted from glands in the body and then transported to where they are needed. Instead, we are able to produce them on the spot in response to a stimulus anywhere in the body. Also unlike hormones, prostaglandins live for only a few seconds before being broken down, which is why we need a steady supply of GLA to ensure our prostaglandin levels remain stable. Chemically speaking, prostaglandins are products of the controlled oxidation of several different highly unsaturated fatty acids. Enzymes are made by the body to oxidise specific essential fatty acids to produce a particular type of prostaglandin. This process of oxidation is very exact, unlike the random and unpredictable process of oxidation in air which produces different substances in uncontrolled amounts.

About thirty different prostaglandins have now been isolated and identified. Each has a highly specific individual function and some have stronger functions than others. The series 1 prostaglandins made from dihomo-gamma-linolenic acid are the best known because they have been subjected to the most detailed study. The most interesting member of the series is E1 or PGE1 which has several important functions in different tissues in the human body. It prevents blood platelets from sticking together and thereby helps prevent heart attacks and strokes caused by blood clots in the arteries. In the kidneys, it helps to remove fluid from the body by acting as a diuretic. It also opens up blood vessels, improving circulation and relieving angina. This particular group of prostaglandins has many other important functions in the body and this is why gamma-linolenic acid is so essential to us as their precursor. The action of prostaglandins as regulators and internal messengers means that they have a dramatic effect on our overall health, and each year literally thousands of medical research papers involving prostaglandin activity are recorded.

Dr Horrobin became so convinced of the amazing possibilities of the GLA in evening primrose oil that he persuaded a director of Agricultural Holdings Ltd to set up another company to research, develop and market evening primrose oil. In 1978 Efamol was formed; as one of the very first companies involved in evening primrose oil it was at the forefront of research into its therapeutic properties. The researchers first discovered that the common factor in most of the conditions such as atopic eczema and diabetes, in which the body is unable to metabolise essential fatty acids correctly, was the reduced activity of the enzyme delta-6-desaturase. It is this enzyme which metabolises the linoleic acid found in food into GLA. A lack of GLA and its metabolites affect the activity of virtually every cell in the body.

The next step was to find a good, stable source of evening primrose oil (there are at least 1,600 varieties of evening primrose). It was also important that the oil be of reproducible quality, as evening primrose oils from different sources contain widely differing quantities of GLA. The wild form of the plant could not be relied upon to produce a consistent quantity and quality of oil and so the Efamol scientists began an extensive programme of plant improvement. All their evening primrose oil products contain a consistent percentage of GLA. Five varieties of Efamol evening primrose plants have been awarded Plant Breeders Rights which is equivalent to a patent in the UK and USA.

Having found a suitable source of evening primrose oil, in-depth clinical studies were set up. The researchers first examined atopic eczema, a common condition especially amongst children. The current conventional treatment is with steroid creams which can affect the immune system and weaken the skin, so a natural remedy with no side-effects would be especially useful. Essential fatty acids (EFAs) play an integral role in all cell membranes and when a patient was fed a diet containing no EFAs, eczema-like skin conditions occurred fairly rapidly. It has been clearly demonstrated that in eczema sufferers, delta-6-desaturase (the enzyme which turns EFAs found in food into GLA) is inactive and so the EFAs are not converted into GLA. The body attempts to overcome this by using other fatty acids which are less effective at maintaining normal skin function.

The causes of pre-menstrual syndrome (PMS) were also researched. An open trial was carried out by Dr Brush at St Thomas's Hospital, London, on sixty-eight women, all of whom had previously failed to respond to other treatment for PMS. The women, many of whom suffered severely from PMS, were prescribed GLA supplements in the form of 500mg capsules of Efamol evening primrose oil. Of the sixty-eight women, 61 percent were said to have experienced total remission from PMS, with a further 23 percent achieving partial remission. Unfortunately, in this first trial, none of the women were given a dummy supplement, or placebo, with which to compare. Dr Horrobin reviewed this trial and three others which were double blind and placebo controlled. The results of these other trials support the supplementation of GLA into the diet of PMS sufferers. One of the trials, which took place in Helsinki, resulted in improvement for 60 percent of women who took the GLA supplement, compared with 40 percent of women who took the placebo or dummy capsule.

Evening primrose oil has also been found to be effective in the treatment of diabetes. In diabetes, the delta-6-desaturase activity is inhibited; taking GLA in the form of evening primrose oil bypasses this process. A report in *The Lancet* in 1986 by Dr Jamal reveals a positive effect of evening primrose oil in reversing diabetic nerve damage in a study of twenty-two patients with diabetic neuropathy who were given 2g of Efamol evening primrose oil capsules twice daily during a six-month double-blind crossover trial.

Other research carried out has revealed that evening primrose oil may be beneficial in many more conditions from alcoholism to certain mental disorders. The quantities of GLA needed to treat any of the above conditions can not be reached through diet alone. We can get enough essential fatty acids through eating polyunsaturated foods but if our delta-6-desaturase is inactive, these will not get converted into GLA. Taking evening primrose oil is more effective than improving the diet, because it bypasses the block caused by delta-6-desaturase inactivity by being a direct source of GLA. Basically, it saves the body the bother of converting oil into a more useful substance.

Another of the richest known sources of GLA is human breast milk – as long as the mother is not atopic (having an inherited susceptibility to certain diseases including eczema and asthma). This is one of the many good reasons for breast feeding your baby as powdered formula milks do not contain added GLA. Breast milk is renowned for its nourishment and ability to protect the immune system. Breast-fed babies are widely known to be better protected against disease, and their levels of GLA may play a part in this. In Japan, GLA is routinely added to powdered baby foods to fortify it. As yet this does not happen in the UK. One way to enrich a baby's formula milk is to add a few drops of pure evening primrose oil to each feed.

HOW EVENING PRIMROSE OIL WORKS

Essential fatty acids – found in polyunsaturated foods contain natural linoleic acid which is converted in the body by delta-6-desaturase into GLA (gamma-linolenic acid).

Disrupting factors – diet and disease: a poor diet that does not contain enough essential fatty acids (EFAs), alcohol, pollution, stress, atopic and viral infections can all block the desaturase enzyme activity.

Evening primrose oil – containing linoleic acid and GLA bypasses the blocked desaturase enzyme activity by supplying GLA directly to the body.

GLA – the correct form of essential fatty acids which are vital for all cell membranes and the body can now produce prostaglandins and other important compounds.

The Supplement Story

Today there are several companies who manufacture supplements and there is an ongoing debate as to who manufactures the best evening primrose oil and other products containing GLA. Efamol, who have done most of the research into the oil and its health-giving properties, claim that their products are of a higher quality than the other products available. Since the discovery of the effects of GLA in the body many other oils have become available which contain large quantities of GLA. Borage oil (sometimes known as starflower oil) in particular contains more GLA than evening primrose oil. Efamol claims, though, that it is not the quantity of GLA that is important; as with everything, it is the quality that counts.

According to Efamol's findings, borage oil is more complex than evening primrose oil. It contains more GLA, and less linoleic acid but more of other fatty acids, including erucic acid which in large amounts is reported to have harmful effects. Research has shown that large amounts of erucic acid can cause platelet aggregation which can lead to thrombosis (the formation of a blood clot in a vein or artery). There have also been clinical trials to compare the effects of evening primrose oil, borage oil and blackcurrant, all of which have a high GLA content. In one trial the oils were examined to see how they converted into prostaglandin E1. This particular study showed that evening primrose oil in the form of Efamol was better than the other oils in producing prostaglandin E1. Dr Horrobin of Efamol states that 'this clearly demonstrates that the GLA content of an oil alone is no guide to its biochemical, and therefore clinical effects.' Some other substance in borage and other oils may interfere with the GLA activity.

The other fatty acids present in an oil must also be considered. The saturated fats in an oil may interfere with the polyunsaturated essential fatty acids. Dr Myher in 1977 expressed that the biological activity of evening primrose oil is probably not due solely to the presence of a single active constituent, but may depend on its whole configuration. Evening primrose oil is also high in linoleic acid (72 percent of the oil is linoleic acid) which works with the GLA instead of against it.

Efamol also claim that their method of extraction is of the highest quality and that other manufacturers of evening primrose oil do not have the same experience in extracting the oil and, therefore, their oils are not of such a high standard. Efamol extract their oil using natural solvents and this releases the sterols and phospholipids in the oil which help to preserve it and prevent it from going rancid. Efamol claim that some other manufacturers of evening primrose oil refine the extracted oil using chemicals, a process which destroys these natural preservatives. The conflicting claims made about evening primrose oil can make choosing supplements a very confusing issue. Which evening primrose oil is really best, and what about borage oil which is cheaper? To decide which supplements to buy we need to look at which products have been thoroughly researched –Naudicelle and Efamol are the two most researched supplements of evening primrose oil and both have been used successfully in many clinical trials. It is also important to choose supplements from well-known, reputable companies. All the good quality manufacturers carry out stringent quality-control tests to ensure that the contents of their capsules are pure and effective.

Borage Oil

However, there have also been several successful tests using borage or starflower oil. A test involving guinea pigs fed on borage was reported in *The Lancet* in 1989. This survey on dietary fatty acids and inflammatory diseases revealed that the guinea pigs produced increased quantities of DGLA metabolites which have anti-inflammatory potential and are, therefore, beneficial in treating eczema and other inflammatory conditions. One trial on borage oil in the treatment of rheumatoid arthritis was reported in the *Annals of Internal Medicine* in November 1993. This twenty-four week double-blind, placebo-controlled trial was carried out by three doctors from different universities in America. Thirty-seven patients with rheumatoid arthritis were treated, some of whom were given borage oil in the form of Boracelle capsules manufactured by Bio-Oil Research. The other patients were given a placebo of cotton seed oil. The total daily dose was four capsules taken three times throughout the day. The condition of the patients was tested at the beginning of the trial and at six-week intervals. After the treatment was finished, the patients who were taking the borage oil showed a clinically important reduction in the signs and symptoms of the disease, whereas the condition of those taking the placebo either did not change at all or worsened. The borage oil reduced the number of tender joints by 36 percent and the swollen joint count by 28 percent. This encouraging report reveals that the GLA content of borage oil is clearly very active.

Borage is grown all over Europe and it is easily recognisable in the herb bed by its bright blue flowers and rough greyish-green leaves. During the Middle Ages borage was a popular anti-inflammatory agent and was also used to treat rheumatism and heart disease. The English herbalist Nicholas Culpeper was ahead of his time when he described borage seeds as being useful for 'increasing the milk in women's breasts', as borage has only recently been identified as one of the richest sources of GLA, the essential fatty acid naturally present in breast milk.

As a result of the research into the medicinal effects of evening primrose oil and its essential fatty acids, scientists began to search for other natural sources of GLA. Borage oil contains more than twice as much GLA as evening primrose oil. In fact, borage seeds consist of a staggering 25 percent pure GLA. This supposedly means that we only need half as much borage oil as evening primrose oil to achieve the same effect. This should be good news for consumers because it means swallowing fewer capsules which should, in theory, cost us less. However, borage oil has not yet captured the following that evening primrose oil has. There has been much more investment in extensive research into the medicinal properties of evening primrose oil. Nevertheless, it can only be a matter of time before the extraordinary potential of borage oil is fully tested and recognised. As yet there has been very little research into borage oil, so if you want to be certain that you will receive all the benefits of GLA outlined in this *Quick Guide*, then it is perhaps better to buy evening primrose oil. You can of course carry out your own trial on borage oil by testing its powers on yourself.

It is now common knowledge amongst biochemists that GLA is needed for many bodily functions, and that it can be created by the body from the linoleic acid commonly found in nuts, seeds and vegetables. However, we also know that this conversion process may be blocked by many factors of modern living, including internal pollution from smoking, external pollution from chemicals (such as car fumes), and stress. The average Western diet is full of saturated fats, processed foods and alcohol all of which affect the important conversion of linoleic acid into GLA. As a result, many of us now risk deficiency of GLA. So if you suffer from atopic eczema, premenstrual syndrome, or any of the other conditions associated with lack of GLA, then try changing your diet, at least temporarily, to see if the condition improves. Also consider taking evening primrose oil capsules or other supplements from reputable manufacturers made with GLA. Don't be tempted to buy low-price supplements from dubious sources – as with most things in life, you tend to get what you pay for.

A Guide to Dosage

Different people may require different doses of evening primrose oil or other GLA supplements to feel any effect. The best dose for the individual may be found by a simple process of trial and error to see what works. Evening primrose oil has very few side-effects even when taken in large doses so it is perfectly safe to experiment with the dosage. In some cases patients have shown side-effects of lethargy or headaches – if this happens simply lower the dose. Another minor side-effect is mild diarrhoea; also, some long-term female users have reported that their breasts have enlarged (some may see this as a benefit, of course). Evening primrose oil may occasionally affect the menstrual cycle, making it longer: from twenty-eight days to thirty-one or thirty-two days or even longer. Drs Nazzaro and Lombard in the USA have also found that it can make people feel forgetful. These doctors were getting an overall 70 percent success rate in cases of pre-menstrual syndrome (PMS) on doses as low as one or two capsules of 500mg evening primrose oil a day. In contrast, the Women's Nutritional Advisory Service in Hove, East Sussex, found an improvement in 83 percent of women in a trial suffering from PMS who were taking eight 500mg capsules a day. The ideal doses may also vary depending on age and what condition is being treated.

Caution: Evening primrose oil should not be taken by anyone with temporal lobe epilepsy.

Evening primrose oil works best when it is taken with other nutrients which help in the metabolism of essential fatty acids. These are:

* Vitamin C
* Vitamin B6
* Nicotinamide (vitamin B3) or niacin
* Zinc
* Magnesium.

Evening primrose oil should always be taken with vitamin E which acts as an antioxidant and prevents the oil from going rancid. Many evening primrose oil capsules contain vitamin E but some of the cheaper brands do not. To achieve the best effect from essential fatty acids, the linoleic acid in evening primrose oil should be balanced with an intake of the alpha-linolenic family. These can be best taken in the form of a fish oil capsule and plenty of fresh fish should also be eaten.

In most cases evening primrose oil takes a couple of months before any improvement in severe disorders such as eczema or mastalgia (breast pain) is noticed. It is not a fast-acting drug and the time it takes to start working depends upon the individual taking it and the condition for which they are taking it.

The following doses are those recommended by the Evening Primrose Office, a public information service which collates and distributes the latest medical findings on this supplement.

Eczema	6 x 500mg per day
Hangover	6 x 500mg before drinking
Breast pain	6 x 500mg per day
Pre-menstrual syndrome	2 x 500mg per day (for severe PMS)
	2 x 250mg per day (for mild PMS)
Skin, hair and general health	2 x 250mg per day or 1 x 500mg per day

—2—

Evening Primrose Oil and the Skin

Anti-ageing

Caring for the skin from within is as important, if not more so, than preventing the signs of premature ageing with external skincare. To maintain a glowing, youthful appearance, it is important to nourish your skin. The skin relies on an extensive network of blood vessels for a steady supply of essential nutrients. Unfortunately, the body's blood circulation does not always deliver the goods, and the skin is very sensitive to nutritional deficiencies. This is because other organs in the body take priority, and essential nutrients may be directed to other areas, such as the heart, brain and muscles, leaving the skin short-changed. The only way to keep the dermis healthy and strong is with optimum nutrition and this includes a daily dose of the all-important essential fatty acids, vitamin E and lecithin. Natural plant oils are the very best source of these skin-savers. These vital oils include unrefined sunflower, corn and sesame seed oils for cooking and, of course, evening primrose oil and other GLA supplements. Maintaining healthy-looking, youthful skin is really a case of inner health, outer beauty.

Watching what we eat is a fundamental part of improving dry skin conditions and the visible signs of ageing. Saturated fats are very damaging to dry skin as they block the body's natural conversion of linoleic acid to GLA. Without this essential fatty acid our skin cells weaken, and their protective membranes lose internal moisture. The GLA in evening primrose oil helps strengthen the delicate membranes surrounding skin cells, increasing their chances of resisting attack from destructive enzymes during the ageing process. GLA can also slow the signs of ageing by keeping our skin cells functioning in a healthy way for longer. It can also help cells resist the attacks from free-radicals that lead to cellular disorganisation and an increased risk of cancer and heart disease. GLA is occasionally added to skin cream in the form of evening primrose oil, but its most effective anti-ageing action comes from taking the oil internally. Most capsules containing evening primrose oil also contain vitamin E, an important antioxidant which fights the free-radicals that are so damaging to skin cells. Vitamin E also preserves the evening primrose oil, so it is doubly important.

Skincare

Hormones play a major part in the way our skin behaves and are responsible for pre-menstrual spots, adolescent acne, stretch marks during pregnancy and patches of uneven pigmentation during the menopause. The essential fatty acid GLA, found in evening primrose oil, affects the production of prostaglandins which have a powerful effect on the state of the skin.

DRY SKIN

The nutritional significance of essential fatty acids such as GLA was initially highlighted in trials involving rats fed on a totally fat-free diet. The rats quickly developed skin disorders, most notably very dry, scaling patches of skin. We will also see similar skin disorders if we cut fat and oil from our diets completely, which is one reason why fat-free diets are so damaging. Those following a very low-fat diet often complain of very dry, scaly patches of skin. This leads to premature lines and wrinkles on the face and body.

One of the many functions of the essential fatty acids in our diet is to maintain the water barrier that exists between the stratum corneum, or uppermost layer of skin cells. A dry, devitalised complexion is not caused by lack of oil in the skin, but is due instead to the evaporation of water through this barrier. Therefore any holes or weakened areas in it will allow more moisture to escape and lead to excessively dry skin. GLA is an important constituent of the cellular membranes that make up this barrier, so we need to receive regular supplies to ensure that it remains stable and strong. In the skin as in all organs, essential fatty acids are principally found in phospholipids (oils) and are important for the strength and structure of our cell membranes and enzymes. These fatty acids are highly unsaturated and this makes these structures very fluid.

As has already been shown, an arguably more important function of some of the essential fatty acids (especially GLA), is as a maker of prostaglandins. There have been several hundred reports on the synthesis and role of prostaglandins in the skin over recent years. There is even an orang-utan at London Zoo which has been cured of flaking skin and a lack-lustre coat with a regular dose of evening primrose oil!

While a daily internal dose of evening primrose oil can significantly improve the look and feel of dry skin, the capsules can also be pierced and the contents rubbed into the skin. The GLA in the evening primrose oil will be absorbed by the uppermost layers of skin cells and will help prevent vital moisture loss. Because it is quite sticky, concentrated oil is easiest to use when blended with another lighter oil, such as grapeseed or safflower. This mixture then forms a protective layer on the epidermis and keeps the complexion supple and strong. The mixture will keep for about a month if stored in a cool, dark place, and can be used instead of expensive skin creams or body lotions. The capacity of evening primrose oil to care for the skin has meant that an increasing number of skincare ranges utilise it.

However, because the oil is an expensive ingredient and has a limited shelf life, few creams contain significant quantities. To get the maximum benefit from the oil, I prefer to add the fresh contents of a capsule to a small jar of moisturiser, and use this within a few weeks, making more when required.

Moisture booster face mask: To give your skin an instant 'fix' of moisture, here is a recipe for a face mask which is quick and easy to make. You need the following ingredients:

> *1/2 small ripe avocado*
> *1 egg yolk*
> *5ml (1tsp) olive oil*
> *1 500mg capsule of evening primrose oil*

Mix the avocado, egg yolk, and olive oil together, then pierce the capsule of evening primrose oil and empty it into the mixture. Continue to mix until the ingredients combine to form a smooth paste. Apply this to clean skin on the throat, neck and upper chest area (you may find it easier to use a large make-up brush or pastry brush to paint the face mask on to the skin). Relax for 15–20 minutes to give the emollient ingredients enough time to penetrate the upper levels of the skin. Remove with tissues or dampened cotton-wool pads.

COMBINATION SKIN
Re-balancing the amount of sebum produced by the sebaceous glands in the skin is the most important part of coping with combination skin. As we have seen, saturated fats in the diet block the body's process of converting linoleic acid into GLA which results in an imbalance of prostaglandin activity. This imbalance leads to excessive sebum production, so a daily dose of evening primrose oil can help. GLA also regulates hormonal activity. Hormonal changes occur after taking the contraceptive

pill, becoming pregnant or taking hormone replacement therapy (HRT). A daily dose of GLA may help prevent the results of these unusual imbalances becoming visible in the skin. Far from making the skin more oily, a daily dose of evening primrose oil can help regulate the skin's natural sebum production.

OILY SKIN AND ACNE

Very oily skin and acne are both caused by the same contributing factor: excessive sebum production. Over 70 percent of teenagers are estimated to have acne at any one time, although most of this is classified as mild acne which usually clears up naturally within twelve months. Acne is not only a teenage skin condition, however, and it is not uncommon for it to strike us for the first time when we are in our twenties. The amount of sebum (the skin's natural oil) produced by the sebaceous glands is controlled by a group of male hormones known as androgens. The main androgen responsible for regulating sebum output is testosterone, a hormone found in both men and women. It is an imbalance of testosterone during puberty, or occasionally during pregnancy, that triggers excessive sebum production. The problem with producing too much sebum is that it tends to build up and block the pores and hair follicles. If this happens, bacteria quickly multiply beneath the blockage and inflammation soon sets in. This leads to the formation of pus and the familiar yellow-headed pustule.

There is no doubt that a nutrient-enriched wholefood diet is extremely helpful in improving these skin conditions. It is also extremely important that those with acne avoid all saturated fats. The most important nutrients in our diet are the essential fatty acids which strengthen skin cells, vitamin E for skin healing, lecithin for clearing the build-up of fatty waste matter beneath the skin, and vitamin A and zinc for repairing the skin. Evening primrose oil supplements are a rich source of vitamin

E (which is added to most capsules), the important essential fatty acid GLA and lecithin. Taking evening primrose daily will help to re-balance the sebum production within the skin.

Evening Primrose Oil for All-round Beauty

A balanced diet, enriched by evening primrose oil, is a fundamental factor in preserving your face and warding off wrinkles. However, evening primrose oil does not just benefit the condition of the skin, it is also a natural cosmetic that improves the quality and look of both hair and nails. Research has shown that a deficiency of essential fatty acids results in increased sebum production. Sebum is the hair's natural lubricant but over-production results in greasy hair and a flaking scalp.

The linoleic and gamma-linolenic acid in evening primrose oil also seems to have an ability to strengthen the nails. Many of the women taking part in evening primrose oil trials report that their brittle nail problems dramatically improve during treatment. So even if you are not suffering from a particular medical condition with which evening primrose oil can help, such as eczema, it is still a good idea to take a daily dose to maintain a youthful appearance. In addition, taking evening primrose oil may also help protect the body against the following ailments by providing the essential fatty acids it requires.

ECZEMA

On a personal note, my first encounter with evening primrose oil was more than ten years ago during a particularly bad attack of eczema. I have had a lifetime's experience of this skin disorder and would watch it flare up with depressing regularity during periods of stress or overwork. As a child, my condition was controlled with the standard prescription of steroid-based ointments which can leave the skin thinned, and in many cases, permanently scarred, as well as reducing overall immunity. I was lucky, the eczema only affected my arms and legs, not my face, but other sufferers are not so fortunate. Over the years I tried many alternative therapies, but nothing proved to be a permanent cure and I became resigned to covering up with long-sleeved clothing even in the height of summer.

The word eczema is from the Greek verb 'to boil', a good description of the symptoms of chronically inflamed and intensely itchy skin. There are few conditions more demoralising than serious skin disorders that won't respond to treatment, and I will admit to swallowing my first dose of evening primrose oil shrouded in a cloud of gloom. However, the effect was remarkable. Within days the itching stopped and my skin started to heal. The roughened, scaly patches that covered my arms began to fade, until after just one month they had disappeared altogether. I have since taken supplements containing GLA on a regular basis and my eczema has never returned.

Conventional medicine has yet to find a drug that effectively treats eczema and does not have damaging side-effects, yet this is one of the commonest diseases of the skin. Sufferers are driven to distraction by the overwhelming urge to scratch, which inevitably leads to severe scaling, bleeding and weeping of blisters under the skin. Not only is eczema unsightly, it is also extremely uncomfortable and frustratingly difficult to cure. The commonest form of eczema is atopic eczema, thought to be triggered by allergies, and commonest in families where there is a history of asthma and hay fever. Atopic eczema is due to a faulty immune system which leads to the body being unable to distinguish invading bacteria and viruses from harmless environmental substances such as pollen, house dust and house-dust mite droppings. Conventional medication includes steroid and antihistamine drugs, which may work for some sufferers but do have side-effects and are often disappointingly ineffective. Atopic eczema is commonest amongst young children and Dr David Atherton, paediatric dermatologist at the Hospital for Sick Children, Great Ormond Street, London is in no doubt of the mental as well as physical scars it leaves on the victim. He says 'in some respects it is easier and less distressing to care for a child with leukaemia than a child suffering from atopic eczema. The disease causes unbearable physical distress for which there is often little relief.'

Children who develop atopic eczema usually do so between the ages of three and six months at the time when most are weaned. One clue that the gamma-linolenic acid in evening primrose oil could be a factor in curing eczema was found when breast-fed babies who switched to solids developed the disease. Human breast milk contains GLA and breast-fed babies receive an equivalent amount of GLA as found in two or three capsules of evening primrose oil every day. Although the makers of formula feeds claim their products are as close in composition as possible to human milk, rather surprisingly they do not contain any GLA at all. According to one manufacturer, adding GLA is 'unnecessary and impractical' and would reduce shelf life. However, the Japanese manage to add GLA to their formula milks by a process of micro-encapsulation. British formula milks contain linoleic acid, which should be converted by the body into GLA. However, studies have shown that some babies do not carry out this conversion process properly.

Even solely breast-fed babies may not receive enough GLA to protect them from eczema if their mother's blood has low levels of GLA. It may therefore be sensible for breast-feeding women to supplement their diet with evening primrose oil. Studies show that children already suffering from atopic eczema (the most common kind) have unusually low levels of unsaturated fatty acids in their bloodstream. The news that most of these children will outgrow eczema by the time they reach puberty is of little consolation to those enduring the agonies of it at the time. Some people in middle or later life may also develop eczema, although when they were young adults they appeared to have healthy skin. This later emergence of the skin problem is therefore likely to represent a recurrence of atopic disease. Atopic eczema usually runs in families which suggests that genetics is also involved. As with most conditions, prevention is often easier than a cure, and GLA supplements may be a useful option for those with atopic eczema in the family.

Evening primrose oil can also be applied externally to the affected areas of the skin. Those with eczema should avoid using soap or any kind of foaming detergent-based cleanser on their skin. Other gentle alternatives include the Oilatum and Aveeno therapeutic skincare ranges. Here is a simple but effective recipe for making a skin oil at home:

Eczema skin oil

> 15ml (1tbsp) calendula oil
> 15ml (1tbsp) St John's wort oil
> 5ml (1tsp) wheatgerm oil
> 5ml (1tsp) evening primrose oil

Mix all the oils together and store in an airtight jar away from heat and light. This richly nourishing oil contains important essential fatty acids, vitamin E and several soothing herbal compounds to help relieve the itch and scaling associated with eczema. It is safe to use on babies and children and should be applied to clean, dry skin twice daily.

Evening primrose oil can be bought in a dropper bottle or obtained by squeezing out the contents from a couple of capsules. You can buy calendula oil and St John's wort oil ready-made from herbal or aromatherapy suppliers (see Useful Addresses).

THE PROOF THAT GLA CAN HELP ECZEMA

Having established the link between GLA in evening primrose oil and eczema, literally hundreds of trials involving eczema sufferers have taken place. One of the most widely published was carried out by the Department of Dermatology at Bristol's Royal Infirmary and the results, published in *The Lancet*, report a significant improvement in patients with atopic eczema. These improvements were recorded after just three weeks of taking 4,000mg of evening primrose oil a day (2,000mg a day for children). The evening primrose oil was shown to lessen itching by 36 percent, scaling by 33 percent and redness by 29 percent. Another trial was carried out in the Departments of Physiology and Dermatology at the University of Turku in Finland which was published in the *British Journal of Dermatology* in 1987. Twenty-five young adults (nine males and sixteen females), aged nineteen to thirty-one years, with moderate to severe atopic eczema, were studied. Eighteen of the patients had a family history of atopy. They were divided into two random groups, fourteen patients were given evening primrose oil (Efamol) and eleven were given a placebo, in a double-blind trial, so neither the doctors nor the patients knew who was receiving what. Four 500mg capsules were taken twice daily by the group of fourteen patients while the placebo contained liquid paraffin. The patients were instructed to keep their diet unchanged during the study period and no potent steroids and other drugs were used. The extent and severity of the eczema was assessed at the start of the trial and every three weeks thereafter, always by the same dermatologist. After twelve weeks of treatment all the patients except one in the evening primrose group improved significantly, with the dryness, itch and general surface area of the eczema all significantly reduced, and the level of DGLA (dihomo-gamma-linolenic acid and the precursor to prostaglandin E1) increased in every patient. In contrast, those in the placebo group made only a small improvement, and there was no correlation between the improvement in the severity of the eczema and an increased level of DGLA.

Similar trials at the Dermatology Clinic at the University of Bologna in Italy report 'substantial improvements' in the clinical symptoms of atopic eczema after four weeks of evening primrose oil therapy. The trial was carried out on twelve young children, eight males and four females, aged two to four years, who all suffered from atopic eczema. The children were given six 500mg capsules a day of Efamol evening primrose oil. The clinical results showed that the significant improvement in the children's conditions was maintained after twenty weeks of the therapy.

Evening primrose oil is now available on prescription from your GP for the relief of atopic eczema and, as children often have difficulty swallowing large capsules, it also comes in capsules with a neck that can be snipped off so the oil can be squeezed onto food or into a drink. Its medical name is Epogam and it is a patented form of GLA from pure evening primrose oil. Capsules of evening primrose oil are particularly effective in relieving the 'itch' of eczema and it is the GLA which produces quantities of DGLA (dihomo-gamma-linolenic acid) metabolites which are in turn converted into prostaglandin E1 which is anti-inflammatory and very beneficial to the body. This is how GLA is able to reduce the itching and appearance of lesions due to eczema and other skin conditions.

PSORIASIS

Some psoriasis sufferers also seem to benefit from taking evening primrose oil, although the research is not as conclusive. Some clinical trials report moderate improvements in 60 percent of patients given evening primrose oil over an eight-week period. Eskimos traditionally have a very 'fishy' diet and they tend not to suffer from psoriasis. Fish oils are a good source of essential fatty acids and it has been demonstrated that when eskimos switch to a Western diet with a higher intake of saturated fats, the development of psoriasis is more common. Again, if the essential fatty acids are unable to be converted to GLA, then it is beneficial to supply the body directly with GLA through evening primrose oil capsules.

AIDS

Recent research carried out by Dr Horrobin shows promise of evening primrose oil in alleviating symptoms of AIDS sufferers, such as skin sores and fatigue. The research was carried out in Tanzania and found improvements after AIDS patients took a combination of evening primrose and fish oil in twelve capsules a day for at least three months. This is by no means a cure, but, as Dr Horrobin says, 'the effects appear to reinforce evidence about how essential fatty acids can affect the immune system.' The research also suggests that low EFA levels can stop the body's natural virus killer, interferon, from working. This may help to explain why the laboratory-produced interferon, which was hailed as the wonder drug in the seventies, has never lived up to its promise; the patients who took it may have had low levels of essential fatty acids which may have inhibited the effect of the drug.

Recently there has been an increasing interest in researching new targets for anti-viral chemotherapy, and one particular study has investigated the selective cell-killing effect of the lithium salt in GLA. Some polyunsaturated essential fatty acids have been found to be anti-viral and gamma-linolenyl alcohol was discovered to be a particularly powerful compound. Gamma-linolenic acid was found to be particularly good at selecting infected cells, and a study was set up to investigate the effects of GLA on cells chronically affected with HIV and on cell-to-cell transmission. The study was carried out by a team at the Medical College of St Bartholomew's Hospital in London.

They tested the possibility that lithium gammalinolenate (Li-GLA), which is now being developed by Scotia Pharmaceuticals as a treatment for pancreatic and other cancers, might also be effective on HIV-infected cells. Previous studies have revealed that tumour cells are selectively killed when supplemented with polyunsaturated essential fatty acids, while the normal cells are left unharmed. The study carried out by the group at St Bartholomew's demonstrated that Li-GLA given in vitro (ie in a test-tube) selectively kills cells which are chronically infected with HIV. This is a major breakthrough in the search for a cure for the HIV virus. Further work is being carried out to investigate the properties of Li-GLA in HIV infections, and whether the same results might be reproduced in humans.

3

Evening Primrose Oil and PMS

It is thought that about 40 percent of women worldwide suffer from some form of pre-menstrual syndrome and about 10 percent are thought to experience extreme PMS. Many sufferers first experience the symptoms of irritability and depression during their teens, while others escape until their early thirties. It affects all races and levels of society and some of the more famous sufferers have included Queen Victoria, Maria Callas, Marilyn Monroe and Judy Garland. PMS can cause severe emotional upset. In 1980 two British women, separately accused of murder, pleaded pre-menstrual syndrome as part of their defence. As a result, both had their charges reduced to manslaughter on the grounds of diminished responsibility and were put on probation.

One of the main causes of PMS is the imbalance between the hormones oestrogen, progesterone and prolactin just before menstruation. An excess of prolactin in particular is linked to high stress levels and has a direct effect on breast pain, causing tenderness and swelling. These three hormones are governed by a group of prostaglandins called PGE1, PGE2 and PGF2, which can cause the uterine contractions that lead to stomach cramps and water retention. Most women experience PMS to some degree with a wide variety of unpleasant symptoms including irritability, weight gain, tender breasts, depression, lethargy, cravings for food and drink and even violent tendencies. These mental and physical changes can take place at any time between two and fourteen days before menstruation and are relieved almost immediately before the period starts.

The Contributory Factors of PMS

* Lack of essential fatty acids and prostaglandin E1

* Poor diet containing too much saturated fat, sugar, tea and coffee

* Drugs, alcohol and smoking

* Pollution from petrol fumes, chemical sprays, etc

* The contraceptive pill

* Hormonal imbalances

* Stress

* Pregnancies – PMS can sometimes get worse after a second pregnancy

* Candida albicans, the yeast infection, can either exacerbate PMS or be mistaken for PMS.

Evening primrose oil is known to affect and regulate the action of prostaglandins and has undergone extensive trials to try to pin-point its action in relieving PMS. One such experiment, detailed in the *Pharmaceutical Journal*, took place at St Thomas's Hospital in London. Sixty-eight women were involved, all of whom were classed as having PMS symptoms which had failed to respond to conventional medication. The women were given 2,000mg of evening primrose oil a day (4 x 500mg capsules) and at the end of the trial 61 percent said that they had total relief from PMS, while a further 23 percent reported partial relief. It is thought that the women suffered from low prostaglandin levels caused by poor absorption of linoleic acid or its subsequent conversion into GLA. This is quickly rectified with an evening primrose oil supplement and, by regulating the action of PGE1, PGE2 and PGF2, the oil corrects the imbalances that can lead to PMS in many sufferers.

Another trial carried out by Drs Massil, Brush and O'Brian involved eighty-nine patients. This large trial was significant as it was both double blind and placebo controlled. In the first cycle of the trial, the patients were untreated so that a clear diagnosis of the level of PMS suffered by each could be established. Patients then received either 500mg capsules of evening primrose oil or placebos (dummy capsules) in a randomised, double-blind manner. This consisted of a three-month period of taking evening primrose oil or a placebo, followed by a four-month period with the reverse treatment. The symptoms of depression, irritability, bloating, breast pain, headache and poor co-ordination were assessed daily. Seventy-seven patients completed the trial. Those taking the evening primrose oil showed a marked improvement in symptoms.

The symptoms of PMS can also be partially relieved through diet and exercise. As with most physical and mental ailments it is important to reassess your whole lifestyle. This usually entails cutting down on unhealthy foods, alcohol consumption and taking more exercise. Aerobic and stretching exercises can provide an outlet for the relief of tension and can help to relax tense muscles. It is also best to avoid eating too much dietary fat as this can lead to excess body weight which can put hormones out of balance and therefore increase the symptoms of PMS. More protein should be eaten in the form of seeds, nuts, fish and poultry. During the run-up to their period, many women often experience cravings for sweet food, but these should be curbed where possible, as all sweets and simple sugars can increase moodiness by causing sudden swings in the blood glucose levels. If you are susceptible to water retention then you should limit your salt intake and it is also beneficial to limit your intake of alcohol, caffeine and nicotine in the run-up to your period. For those who prefer to eat little and often as opposed to having a couple of large meals a day, this method of eating may help balance energy levels and help the absorption of nutrients and may help relieve the symptoms of PMS.

Menopause

Evening primrose oil may also be able to help ease the symptoms of the menopause. One common symptom is depression, similar to that experienced by many women before they menstruate. The exact cause of this depression is unknown. However, some of the proposed causes are an imbalance in oestrogen and progesterone levels, extensive swings in hormone levels and prostaglandin imbalances. Other main symptoms are lethargy, aching bones, muscles or limbs, weight gain, mood swings and irrational feelings. The majority of these symptoms are the same as those of PMS which may be alleviated through taking evening primrose oil capsules.

Many women take HRT (Hormone Replacement Therapy) to avoid the unpleasant symptoms. Unfortunately one of the side-effects for some women who previously suffered from PMS is a continuation of symptoms such as breast pain.

Perhaps the most uncomfortable and common symptom of the menopause is hot flushes. It was thought initially that evening primrose oil may be able to help treat this. A double-blind, placebo-controlled trial was carried out to test the effectiveness of evening primrose oil in treating fifty-six menopausal women who suffered from hot flushes at least three times a day. The exact cause of hot flushes is unknown, although it has been suggested that oestrogen deficiency may be to blame. Women taking any form of oestrogen replacement therapy or other drugs for menopausal symptoms were excluded from the study. The trial took place at the North Staffordshire Hospital Centre, Stoke-on-Trent and at the Royal Free Hospital, London and was conducted over seventeen months. Eighteen women given gamma-linolenic acid (GLA) in the form of evening primrose oil, and twenty-eight women taking the placebo completed the trial. In women taking the evening primrose oil the only significant improvement was a reduction in the maximum number of night-time flushes.

Some menopausal symptoms can be psychological and it can be difficult to establish which ones are directly linked to the menopause because women in their late forties and fifties are often experiencing more than their fair share of additional stress. Common family stresses include troublesome teenagers, children or partners leaving home and elderly parents. Career women also have their stresses, perhaps feelings of guilt about neglecting their children or those who have never had any children may suddenly feel a sense of loss. Women who have had children late may find that they have to cope with young children, who demand a lot of attention, when their mental and physical energies are lower than usual. In all these cases, the menopause can come at just the wrong time and therefore its effects are often enhanced by all these other external factors.

When the menopause does eventually take effect not all women experience the same symptoms or to the same degree. It is interesting to note that not all women experience menopausal flushes or sweating. The prevalence of these symptoms is subject to wide cultural differences. There is a higher incidence in Western women than in women from developing countries, who generally seem to suffer fewer complaints. This may have more to do with lifestyle than with anything else. When women reach menopause their basic role in society is changed, they are no longer able to procreate. In most 'primitive' societies, women who have reached menopause have a specific place in society, whereas in Western culture menopausal women are perceived as no longer having any particular role to play. In most developing countries women are expected to assume responsibility for their younger relations. They have special roles within their community as midwives, healers, holy women and a whole range of other responsibilities. For example, Maori women become formal mourners at funeral rites and instruct the younger women in traditional arts and crafts, as well as take part in ritual ceremonies. These new-found roles these women are given after the menopause give them a definite status, and they are probably too busy with their new lives to feel the effects of this hormonal change in the same way that Western women do.

Breast Pain

Pre-menstrual breast tenderness is another complaint that responds well to treatment with evening primrose oil and patients suffering from mastalgia (severe breast pain) can now obtain the oil on prescription from their doctor in a form called Efamast. (Evening primrose oil is one of the few natural products to receive a medical licence and it can be obtained on prescription for both eczema and mastalgia.) Many breast conditions are governed by the action of hormones and breast growth is stimulated during the teenage years by hormonal activity during puberty.

By their early twenties, most women have reached their final bust size, although almost all will notice slight changes in breast shape and texture during their monthly cycle. It is quite common for breasts to enlarge in the two weeks before a period, and to return to normal after the period begins. A much more visible change takes place during pregnancy, when hormones can double breast size and increase blood flow by 180 percent. While these hormone fluctuations are perfectly normal, some trigger other breast problems. The most common breast disorder is pre-menstrual mastalgia which affects some five million women in Britain between the ages of twenty and fifty. Other benign (non-cancerous) breast problems include nodularity or lumpiness in the breast just before a period, and fibroadenoma, a smooth moveable lump most often seen in young women. But breast pain is the commonest complaint and can affect part or all of the breast and even extend to the upper arms.

Although women with breast pain appear to have normal hormone levels, their breast tissues are unusually sensitive to hormonal actions. This increased sensitivity is linked to the pattern of essential fatty acids in the bloodstream and these women often have low levels of GLA. They may also have high levels of saturated fats that increase the effects of hormones on breast tissues and trigger pain. The first experience of mastalgia can cause the terrible fear of breast cancer. Fortunately, breast pain is rarely a symptom of cancer and is also far easier to treat. However, conventional medications are far from ideal. Painkillers and diuretics are frequently ineffective and hormone-related drugs carry their own side-effects.

In an attempt to find a more acceptable, natural cure for breast pain, double-blind clinical trials involving evening primrose oil were carried out at the Breast Clinic of the University of Wales. Here, a pharmaceutical-quality evening primrose oil (Efamast) was compared to the most commonly prescribed drugs, bromocriptine and danazol. All three medications were similarly effective, but their levels of side-effects differed enormously. Only 2.2 percent of those given the evening primrose oil experienced any side-effects at all, compared to 23.6 percent and 24.7 percent for bromocriptine and danazol respectively. Also, the side-effects for those taking the evening primrose oil formulation were much less acute, the most common being a mild stomach upset. The medical team from the Cardiff clinic reported in *The Lancet* that, after reassurance about cancer, the evening primrose oil treatment should be the first line of treatment for breast pain. Their studies found that 45 percent of patients suffering from persistent, severe breast pain benefited from a 3,000mg dose of evening primrose oil. However, as the oil works by changing the essential fatty acid composition of cell membranes it is inevitably a slow cure, and the dose must be taken every day for three to six months.

The Cardiff group also showed that the plasma and red cells of women with breast pain exhibit different fatty acid compositions when compared to normal women. Women with breast pain have more saturated fats and less polyunsaturated (essential) fatty acids than normal individuals. This deficit in polyunsaturated fatty acids applied particularly to gamma-linolenic acid and its derivatives. A change took place in the plasma and red cell fatty acid compositions in women who were treated with evening primrose oil for four months. Their plasma and red cell fatty acid compositions became almost normal.

A word about breast cancer: While evening primrose oil can be effective at treating breast pain, it should not be seen as a panacea for all breast problems. Breast cancer is the biggest cause of cancer deaths in women and so it is vitally important not to confuse benign breast conditions with a potential malignancy. Breast cancer is almost non-existent among those under the age of twenty-five, but once past this age the number of sufferers rises rapidly. Monthly self-examination is important for all women and any lump or change in appearance must be checked by a doctor. It is very scary discovering a breast lump, but the vast majority are benign cysts which are easily removed.

Fluid-filled cysts are simply drained with a fine needle and are not thought to be related in any way to breast cancer.

Weight Loss

Those keeping an eye on their weight and worried about dieting, should bear in mind that significant amounts of calories can be saved by cutting down on saturated fats. It is, though, very important that those on a low-fat diet do not cut out fat completely. We all need our essential fatty acids for the good health of every cell in the body. Oil supplements such as evening primrose oil and cod liver oil contain approximately five calories per capsule, and so they can be allowed on even the strictest regime.

Evening primrose can be a boost to anyone's weight-loss diet because it increases the metabolic rate. This discovery was made completely by chance during a trial on evening primrose for schizophrenia. At Bootham Park Hospital in York it was discovered that several patients who were more than 10 percent over their ideal body weight actively lost weight while taking evening primrose oil. However, the oil had no effect on the weight of those who were within 10 percent of their ideal body weight.

There is another substance which plays a key role in weight loss, brown fat, which is found mainly in the back of the neck and along the backbone. The brown fat does not convert calories into energy for body movement; it burns fat only to produce heat. One of its roles is to stabilise weight and to adapt the body to cold weather. When it works properly, brown fat burns up any excess calories, but when it does not, the fat is stored in the body and causes obesity. The gamma-linolenic acid in evening primrose oil has been found to have a stimulating effect on brown fat tissue. The effects of evening primrose oil were investigated in ten obese patients on a normal diet, against eight obese patients on a calorie-restricted diet. Six weeks later, the evening primrose oil group had lost an average of 5 kilograms, while those on a calorie-controlled diet had lost 6.5 kilograms. The most effective dose was eight capsules a day, but evening primrose oil must not be looked upon as miracle cure for the overweight. This particular trial was only shown to be effective in treating obese people and not the average person who just needs to lose a few pounds.

——4——
Evening Primrose Oil and Rheumatoid Arthritis

Perhaps the most exciting development in the use of evening primrose oil has been in its effect on rheumatoid arthritis. Many sufferers of the disease have been able to reduce their dosage of non-steroidal anti-inflammatory drugs, and some have given them up completely thanks to evening primrose oil. Rheumatoid arthritis is a very common disorder (one in twenty people in Britain are affected at some time in their lives) in which the joints in the fingers, wrists, feet, ankles, hips and shoulders become inflamed. Some people may be severely crippled by the disease and it does not only affect the elderly.

Evening primrose oil is sometimes effective in treating the condition because it acts as a precursor to prostaglandins. To put things simply, people who suffer from rheumatoid arthritis have too many of the wrong kind of prostaglandins. These are the series 2 prostaglandins which have an inflammatory effect. Evening primrose oil produces series 1 prostaglandins which are anti-inflammatory. But there is another very important group of biological regulators called leukotrienes, which also have their origin in essential fatty acids. These substances can have an anti-inflammatory effect on the body. Linoleic acid, in the form of fish oils, gets converted into arachidonic acid and this in turn gets converted into leukotrienes. Like prostaglandins, leukotrienes have a startling variety of effects, some of which are very good while others can be harmful.

Leukotrienes help to regulate inflammatory disorders and the level of these regulators in the body must be carefully balanced. Too many leukotrienes can result in them instructing cells to begin harmful disease processes such as blood clots and inflammation. Cod liver oil is able to regulate the leukotrienes, making it a very useful supplement in the battle against inflammatory disorders such as arthritis.

One of the best-known cod liver oil enthusiasts of this century was American laboratory technician Dale Alexander, otherwise known as 'The Cod Father'. His passion for this amber nectar stemmed from the fact that it cured his mother's painful arthritis, and *Arthritis and Common Sense* was the first of five books he wrote on the subject. Alexander advocated a tablespoon of cod liver oil a day mixed with milk to disguise what he called its three flavours, 'ucky, yucky and bloody awful'. The first scientific paper published on cod liver oil and arthritis appeared in a 1959 edition of *The Journal of the National Medicine Association*. This described a study where ninety-eight patients were given 20ml of cod liver oil mixed with milk or orange juice, taken on an empty stomach. A 92 percent success rate in relieving pain and swelling was recorded, with many patients also noticing improved hair, skin and nail condition.

Evening primrose oil does not convert into leukotrienes because dihomo-gamma-linolenic acid cannot give rise to leukotrienes. However, evening primrose oil can help protect the body from the more harmful effects of leukotrienes. It works as an anti-inflammatory agent because prostaglandin E1 works like steroid drugs by blocking the conversion of arachidonic acid into leukotrienes. Tests have shown that mice which have developed arthritis have an increased lifespan when treated with evening primrose oil. It has also been shown to relieve inflammation.

A study was carried out at Glasgow Royal Infirmary involving forty-nine patients with rheumatoid arthritis. Sixteen of the patients were given evening primrose oil in the form of Efamol, fifteen were given a combination of evening primrose oil and fish oil (Efamol Marine), and eighteen were given a placebo. This study set out to establish whether evening primrose oil or evening primrose oil combined with fish oil could replace the conventional non-steroidal anti-inflammatory drug (NSAID) treatment in rheumatoid arthritis. The treatment lasted for fifteen months, but after twelve months all the patients were given a placebo. The patients took three tablets four times daily, and none of the patients knew which treatment they were having. After twelve months the patients taking Efamol and Efamol Marine (with added fish oils) had significantly reduced their NSAIDs intake. This reduction in drug intake did not make the disease get any worse. Sixty percent of the patients who took evening primrose oil on its own were able to stop taking the drugs completely, and a further 25 percent were able to halve their doses without any harmful effects. However, the best results were for the group who took Efamol Marine. Sixty percent of these patients were able to stop taking all anti-inflammatory drugs, while 35 percent halved their doses. Finally, all the patients were given a placebo during the last three months of the trial, and all but one patient suffered a relapse.

This is clearly very good news for all arthritis sufferers because evening primrose is a natural product with no harmful side-effects, whereas NSAIDs do have side-effects. Most NSAIDs reduce the formation of prostaglandins, not only the series 2 prostaglandins which are inflammatory, but also the anti-inflammatory series 1 prostaglandins. In contrast, evening primrose oil prevents the production of series 2 prostaglandins, and harmful leukotrienes, but at the same time it creates the beneficial series 1 prostaglandins and achieves a good balance.

5

Evening Primrose Oil and Multiple Sclerosis

Multiple sclerosis (MS) affects one in a thousand people in Britain and most of its sufferers are young adult women. Although the exact cause of MS is not yet known, it is believed to be an auto-immune disorder, triggered when the body's own immune system starts attacking itself. The disease affects the nervous system and begins with the destruction of the protective sheath called myelin that surrounds nerve fibres in the brain and spinal cord. The symptoms of MS include blurred vision and a tingling or numbness in the body which can lead to paralysis in later life. These symptoms vary in severity and may come and go from one week to the next, so a patient who is severely disabled one week may seem quite normal the next.

While it is not known what prompts MS to strike, those with MS do lack certain essential fatty acids, especially linoleic acid. This deficiency is thought to be an important factor in the degenerative nature of the disease. Studies using evening primrose oil have found its high levels of GLA useful in preventing the immune system's white blood cells from attacking the myelin sheath and destroying the vulnerable nerve cells underneath. In MS, the T-suppressor lymphocytes (white blood cells) which keep the other parts of the immune system under control are thought to be defective. When T-suppressor cells are defective auto-immune damage frequently occurs and prostaglandin E1 may help prevent this. The GLA in evening primrose oil is a precursor to prostaglandin E1 which is also known to strengthen blood vessel walls. This is particularly important in MS with growing evidence that blood vessel walls are breached allowing blood – which is toxic to nerve tissue – to seep into the brain. It is important that blood vessel walls are strengthened to make them withstand clumps of platelets and cholesterol sticking to the walls. The red blood cells of MS sufferers are very low in essential fatty acids and are also much bigger than is normal and are consequently not very effective in regulating the passage of fluids through cell membranes.

Evening primrose oil can correct this problem in a matter of months. One follow-up trial involving evening primrose oil was reported in *The Lancet* in May 1979. MS patients were on long-term treatment with evening primrose oil (Naudicelle) and were also following a diet low in saturated fat. It was found that the mobility of red cells returned to normal. Some medics suggest that evening primrose oil may help more active children suffering from MS, and that it may help if given as a protective measure to children in MS families.

Throughout the 1970s many patients with MS began to take evening primrose oil although it was not until 1978 that the first trial involving evening primrose oil in the treatment of MS was carried out by Professor David Bates in Newcastle. One hundred and sixteen patients with MS were divided into four groups. One group was given evening primrose oil in the form of Naudicelle capsules (six taken daily) and one group was given olive oil in capsules. Another group was given Flora sunflower margarine to eat as a spread and one group was given another spread. None of the patients were aware of which treatment they were having. After two years there was no significant difference in disability between any of the groups. However, the best results were in the group who took the Flora sunflower seed oil spread: the duration and severity of their attacks were less severe.

At first it was thought that the trial demonstrated that evening primrose oil is not effective in treating MS. However,

Dr Dworkin, who later re-examined the case, made a very important discovery – patients who had very low levels of disability at the start of the trial did not get any worse after two years of taking polyunsaturates. One of the reasons why evening primrose oil did not prove to be effective in this trial was that the dose was not high enough. Another interfering factor was that the Naudicelle capsules used at the time had coloured shells (orange and black) which used the food dye tartrazine. It is now known that tartrazine interferes with fatty acid metabolism and so evening primrose oil capsules are now produced in clear, gelatin capsules. Sadly, no more clinical trials of evening primrose oil in the treatment of MS have been carried out since. Evening primrose oil is not prescribable on the NHS as a treatment for MS and many people with MS find buying the capsules too expensive and so do not bother.

MS – A Case History

Sue was twenty-nine when multiple sclerosis struck. A previously healthy, energetic and athletic person, her first symptoms were blurred vision and dizziness. 'I woke up one morning and realised that my eyes wouldn't focus properly. When I stood up I felt very dizzy and unsteady, and I couldn't control my eyes. My neurologist recommended taking evening primrose oil from the beginning. It was also recommended by my doctor, who luckily for me is one of the more enlightened medics. I was diagnosed in May 1988, and have been taking six capsules a day ever since (each containing 430mg evening primrose oil and 107mg fish oil). I have to touch wood before I say that my symptoms have never returned and I can honestly say that I have never felt healthier. I have totally reassessed my diet and don't ever eat any saturated fat. All my oil require-

ments come from the evening primrose capsules. I think that you've just got to start thinking about making the cellular insulation material myelin. Taking evening primrose oil provides the essential fatty acids from the body in the form of GLA which is like giving fat in a pre-digested form. I'm sure that if I stopped taking it my cells would be less protected and I won't take that risk. I feel much better now altogether – my cellulite has vanished and my skin has a much smoother, more youthful texture. I put it down to my revised diet and would advise any sufferer to seek advice from an informed doctor or qualified nutritionist.'

Essential fatty acids are needed by the body to produce myelin, the nerve sheath which breaks down in MS, but which can be regenerated. Evening primrose oil contains the essential fatty acid GLA which produces the prostaglandin E1. This all-powerful prostaglandin is not only responsible for strengthening cell membranes, it also affects the action of nerves. It can produce profound changes in both the central nervous system and the peripheral nervous system. Another of evening primrose oil's many hidden powers is its ability to maintain a healthy balance between the series 1 and 2 prostaglandins. When the body is lacking in essential fatty acids, there is a sudden rise in the series 2 prostaglandins which are made from arachidonic acid. A high level of the series 2 prostaglandins is a symptom of various inflammatory disorders, such as rheumatoid arthritis and possibly MS too. It has been shown that cerebrospinal fluid taken from MS patients contains high levels of prostaglandin F2alpha. Evening primrose oil produces prostaglandin E1 thereby ensuring that a healthy balance is reached between series 1 and 2 prostaglandins.

What People With MS Say

Two surveys have been carried out to find out how MS sufferers responded to treatment with evening primrose oil. One was carried out by Bio-Oil Research Ltd (who manufacture Naudicelle) and the other was carried out by ARMS (Action for Research into Multiple Sclerosis). The Bio-Oil Research survey involved 480 people with MS of whom 65 percent felt there had been some improvement in their condition; 43 percent felt that their condition had remained stable; 22 percent said that there had been fewer and less severe attacks; 20 percent said that specific symptoms had been alleviated; and 13 percent reported an improvement in general health. Those who felt that the treatment had made 'some improvement' mentioned the following benefits of taking evening primrose oil:

* Increased mobility

* Increased walking ability

* Reduced spasm

* Improved eyesight

* Improved bladder function

* Relief of constipation

* Improved condition of hair and skin

* Improvement in wound healing

* Regaining correct weight

* Heavy periods returned to normal.

The ARMS survey which involved 177 completed question-naires was equally encouraging: 127 of the MS sufferers said that they had improved while thirty-three reported no change and seventeen felt that their symptoms had worsened. The ARMS members were also asked how long they had been taking evening primrose oil and their answers revealed that improvements increased when they had been taking the capsules for more than four months.

—— 6 ——
Evening Primrose Oil and Diabetes

Diabetes is caused by the body's inability to utilise carbohydrates or sugary foods as the pancreas is not able to make sufficient insulin and so the sugar accumulates instead of being used as energy. The kidneys endeavour to excrete the excess sugar with the result that diabetics also pass more urine than is normal. Diabetics are treated with insulin and must monitor their dietary intake very carefully, strictly monitoring their intake of all refined carbohydrates and alcohol. People suffering from diabetes can encounter complications even when the disease is controlled by insulin and diet. Damage can occur to the heart and circulation, to the eyes, the kidneys and the nerves. This damage to the nerves is known medically as diabetic neuropathy and this can lead to loss of sensation through the skin, skin disorders, muscle weakness, bladder and intestinal problems and even impotence in men.

Clinical tests have revealed that in diabetics the conversion of linoleic acid into gamma-linolenic acid is impaired. The linoleic acid which we get through eating polyunsaturated foods passes through a series of steps of desaturation inside the body. This process produces two useful metabolites which act as precursors to prostaglandins: dihomo-gamma-linolenic acid (DGLA) and arachidonic acid (AA), both of which play important roles in relation to the peripheral nerves. They regulate the balance of platelet aggregation (which can cause thrombosis) through producing the prostaglandin E1 and they also maintain healthy blood flow. The desaturation process which converts dietary linoleic acid into gamma-linolenic acid is blocked in diabetics and so the prostaglandin E1 is not produced. This block may be an important factor in the development of long-term complications in diabetes. However, it can be overcome by supplying diabetics directly with GLA.

Linoleic acid (found in polyunsaturated foods)

↓

Delta-6-desaturase (this converts the linoleic acid into GLA but it is impaired in diabetes)

↓

GLA (gamma-linolenic acid)

↓

Dihomo-gamma-linolenic acid – DGLA (converted GLA)

↓

Arachidonic acid (converted DGLA)

↓

Prostaglandin E1

Several studies have demonstrated the value of GLA supplementation in controlling diabetic cataract, diabetic retinopathy and diabetic cardiovascular complications. Diabetic retinopathy is the most common cause of blindness in middle-aged people. Diabetes can create swellings in the walls of the arteries which feed the retina, causing many tiny haemorrhages, and the retinal tissue disintegrates and dies. In the 1950s Peifer and Holmen demonstrated that diabetic animals required much higher than normal amounts of linoleic acid in their diet to remain healthy. More than a decade later tests were carried out in Argentina by Dr Brenner. He reported that in liver microsomes from diabetic animals there was a reduced rate of conversion of linoleic acid into GLA, leading to low levels of GLA metabolites. It was not until twenty years later that the suggestion was made that some of the complications of human diabetes might be prevented or reversed by bypassing the impaired 6-desaturation step by direct administration of GLA. Clinical trials have revealed that when GLA was fed to diabetic animals in the form of evening primrose oil, levels of dihomo-gamma-linolenic acid increased which reveals that the GLA in evening primrose oil bypasses the 6-desaturation block.

Diabetes in Humans

There is less direct evidence relating to the effect of GLA in humans suffering from diabetes. It is not possible to examine the metabolism of GLA in liver tissue samples and so most of the studies have been more indirect. Recent studies reveal that diabetics who suffer from diabetic neuropathy respond to treatment with GLA in the same way as animals. A randomised, double-blind, placebo-controlled trial was carried out by Drs Carmichael, Lowe and Manku. They studied the effects of evening primrose oil in the treatment of forty-two patients with diabetes. Twenty-seven of the patients suffered from diabetic neuropathy and fifteen had cardiovascular complications. Their ages ranged from twenty-one to eighty-one years and none of the patients abused drugs or admitted heavy alcohol consumption or received any medication other than their usual treatment for diabetes. The clinical trial lasted six months and the

patients received either twelve 500mg capsules of evening primrose oil per day (three capsules four times daily), or an indistin-
guishable placebo, or dummy capsule.

The results of the trial, compared with normal values taken
from twelve age-matched normal subjects, did not show any
difference in cardiovascular risk factors, such as high cholesterol
and blood pressure. However, the trial revealed that at the end
of the six months of treatment, there was a highly significant rise
in dihomo-gamma-linolenic acid in the patients taking the
evening primrose oil. It is this dihomo-gamma-linolenic acid
which is the precursor to prostaglandin E1 which, as we have
seen, is very important for practically every cell in the body.
Evening primrose oil was found to significantly improve the
conditions of patients with diabetic neuropathy. The development of neuropathy has also been shown to reverse in diabetic
patients in other trials, one of which involved 100 people.

A much larger multi-centre trial of the use of gamma-
linolenic acid in diabetic neuropathy was also set up. The first
year was randomised, double blind and placebo controlled.
Then in the second year, unknown to the patients but known to
the doctors, all the patients who wished to continue were
assigned to active treatment. The treatment was twelve 500mg
capsules of evening primrose oil a day and identical placebo
capsules containing liquid paraffin. In the first year the group
taking evening primrose oil had better results on every parame-
ter than the placebo group. One hundred and eleven patients
were involved in the study, fifty-four in the active group and
fifty-seven in the placebo group. The results of the study at
twelve months as compared to six months indicates that trials of
evening primrose oil in diabetic neuropathy should continue
for at least a year. It is also important that patients with diabetes
control their diabetes effectively as this affects the efficiency of
the GLA. Patients who are reasonably well controlled are more
likely to do well in these clinical trials than those who are not.

DIABETIC RETINOPATHY

The degeneration of the retina of the eye is a common complication for diabetics and is also the most common cause of blindness in middle-aged people. It is a result of the diabetes causing swellings in the walls of the arteries which feed the retina. In a placebo-controlled pilot study, gamma-linolenic acid was investigated for its effects on diabetic retinopathy. As has already been shown, diabetics are unable to convert linoleic acid into GLA. This may play a part in the development of diabetic retinopathy. Patients diagnosed as having diabetic retinopathy were either given evening primrose oil or an identical placebo for a period of six months on a double-blind basis. Those patients given evening primrose oil were given six 6g evening primrose oil capsules daily. After the six months, all patients were given evening primrose oil although they were not aware of it and they were studied for a further six months.

In order to establish the results of the treatment all the patients were photographed and were assessed independently by two experienced readers of retinal photographs. Of the ten assessments made in the evening primrose oil group, seven patients showed improvement and three showed no change after the first six months of treatment. Of the twelve assessments in the placebo group, four showed improvement, three showed no change and five actually deteriorated. After twelve months the results improved further: the ten patients taking evening primrose oil all showed significantly higher signs of improvement. In the group of patients who switched to taking evening primrose oil after six months of taking the placebo, seven showed improvement, three showed deterioration and two showed no change.

After the twelve months of treatment all twenty-two patients were followed up. Fourteen showed deterioration on stopping the treatment, one showed no change and seven showed improvement. It is interesting that in the group which received the placebo first and then switched to evening primrose oil after six months, ten out of twelve patients had deteriorated at the follow up while, in the other group which received evening primrose oil throughout, only four out of ten patients showed deterioration. Although this pilot trial did not involve many patients, it gives clear evidence that as a result of taking evening primrose oil there was a trend towards improvement in patients suffering from diabetic retinopathy.

Other trials have been carried out using evening primrose oil combined with fish oils. The two are combined because diabetes blocks the conversion of two families of essential fatty acids, linoleic acid and alpha-linoleic acid. In diabetics the enzyme which converts linoleic acid into gamma-linolenic acid and the enzyme which converts alpha-linoleic acid into eicos-apentaenoic acid are both blocked. These essential fatty acids are eventually converted into important prostaglandins which enable our cells to work in the right way. Evening primrose oil and fish oil supplements bypass both these blockages.

——— 7 ———
Evening Primrose Oil and Alcoholism

Another of evening primrose oil's many uses is the possible prevention of liver failure due to alcoholism. It can also help prevent the dreadful withdrawal symptoms which alcoholics go through when they give up alcohol. For those who are more careful with their drinking but enjoy the odd celebratory drink, evening primrose oil can prevent you from experiencing a hangover the following morning. Again, it is the unsaturated essential fatty acids in evening primrose oil which are responsible for this amazing ability. Previously, salted pickled herring, which contains highly unsaturated fatty acids, was used in Europe for this purpose, but evening primrose oil is more effective. There has even been evidence to suggest that evening primrose oil may be able to help reverse some of the brain damage caused by alcoholism. The conversion of evening primrose oil into prostaglandin E1 assists in treating alcoholism. Alcohol has a paradoxical effect on prostaglandin E1; drinking a small amount of alcohol stimulates the production of prostaglandin E1 but when large amounts of alcohol are consumed the body is robbed of this vitally important prostaglandin.

There have been reports which suggest that drinking small amounts of alcohol is actually good for you. Recent research in North America and Western Europe consistently revealed that the risk of heart disease is reduced in people with a modest intake of alcohol (meaning one or two glasses of wine or a beer or one glass of some kind of spirit a day). This is no excuse to go out drinking heavily, and it is important that all alcohol consumption is kept to a minimum. People who drink at this level are also said to live longer than both teetotallers and those who drink moderate to heavy amounts of alcohol.

Most people drink because it makes them feel good and this may be a result of rising levels of prostaglandin E1. This particular prostaglandin can create euphoric states and doctors have observed euphoric reactions in patients being given intravenous infusion of prostaglandin E1. Other studies carried out on people who feel abnormally euphoric show that they produce more prostaglandin E1 than normal. This euphoric state only comes from drinking small amounts of alcohol. When the level of alcohol is increased a reverse effect occurs. It boosts the conversion of dihomo-gamma-linolenic acid (DGLA) into prostaglandin E1. This seems like a good thing, but it is in fact disastrous because the alcohol stimulates the synthesis of prostaglandin E1 and so draws on the body's limited stores of dihomo-gamma-linolenic acid. When the effects of the alcohol have worn off, the stores of DGLA are often so reduced that the levels of prostaglandin E1 fall below normal.

A moderate to large amount of alcohol is also one of the main blocking agents in the metabolic pathway of essential fatty acids. The alcohol blocks the delta-6-desaturase enzyme, which converts linoleic acid into GLA, and the delta-5-desaturase enzyme which converts DGLA into arachidonic acid. However, it is fascinating that alcohol has no effect on these enzymes when consumed in small amounts.

As a consequence of drinking too much alcohol, no matter how much linoleic acid you eat in your diet, the depleted stores of DGLA cannot be returned to normal. It is thought that many of the effects of alcohol may be related in some way to very low levels of essential fatty acids. The drastic fall in prostaglandin E1 which happens in alcoholism may account for the hangovers, withdrawal symptoms and depression that so often go with heavy drinking. This may also have other serious consequences including an increased risk of heart attacks and strokes, high blood pressure, liver damage and poor efficiency in coping with infections as well as brain and nerve deterioration. Heavy consumption of alcohol affects not just the liver, but our whole appearance through the skin. No matter what your tipple is, all types of alcohol encourage internal dehydration, it should be avoided by those whose skin is the slightest bit dry or sensitive. Those with normal, combination or oily skin types should at least make sure they match every alcoholic drink with an equal amount of water. Alcohol also dilutes the fragile blood vessels in the face, encouraging the tiny capillaries to expand and burst. Much of the network of broken red veins on the cheeks can be attributed to alcohol. Skin rashes are often triggered by the additives or chemical colourants routinely added to wine and liqueur, and virtually all wine contains sulphur dioxide which is also known to cause skin blotchiness. All of this damage caused by alcohol can be minimised by drinking plenty of water or diluted fruit juice and taking 500mg of evening primrose oil before going to bed.

If you are going to a party or an important celebration and you know in advance that you will probably be having a few more alcoholic drinks than you usually do, then take an evening primrose oil capsule before you go out to help prevent some of the damage. This should also prevent you from getting too bad a hangover the morning after. Following these suggestions, so long as you enjoy only the odd drink and do not indulge in heavy alcohol consumption frequently, you should feel only good effects.

—— 8 ——

Evening Primrose Oil
and Schizophrenia

This severe mental disorder affects many people in their teenage years and can completely destroy their lives. It is genetically linked, and if members of your family are schizophrenic there is a greater risk of it happening to you. It also seems to be brought on by stress; one girl I knew, who never coped with stress very well, was under particular pressure during the final examinations of her university degree. She was unable to sleep, eat properly and was continuously convinced that she had left the cooker on at home and had to keep going back to check. Outside pressure from her family to do well in her exams did not help the situation. She managed to complete her exams but almost as soon as they were over, her thoughts became more strange, as did her behaviour, and she was diagnosed as being schizophrenic. As it turned out, she did very well in her final examinations, but I can't help wondering whether if she had not been under such stress her mind would not have been affected so severely.

Schizophrenia is characterised by a disintegration of the process of thinking, of contact with reality and of emotional responsiveness. The patient often experiences delusions and even hallucinations, especially of voices, and becomes socially withdrawn. There is no cure for schizophrenia and when a friend, relative or loved-one develops the disorder, there is very little you can do to help. The patient may suddenly behave very aggressively towards someone very close to them for no logical reason. This is, naturally, extremely upsetting and frustrating for both people involved. There are some drugs that can be used to suppress some of the worst elements of the disorder, but once someone has been diagnosed as having schizophrenia, he or she will never be able to act and respond in the same way as everyone else ever again.

The search for new ways to treat this terrible mental disorder continues, but it has been discovered that evening primrose oil has a significant effect on certain aspects of schizophrenia. Schizophrenics have abnormal amounts of essential fatty acids (EFAs) as do many alcoholics, hyperactive children and those suffering from depression. The EFAs make up around 20 percent of the dry weight of the brain and peripheral nerves. These EFAs are unlike those present in other body tissues; nearly all those present in nerve tissue have gone through the delta-6-desaturation process, which means the process is even more important in the brain than in any other area in the body. Schizophrenics are low in the series 1 prostaglandins and high in the series 2 prostaglandins. It is not known why these abnormalities exist, but they seem to be partially linked to abnormalities in the precursors to these prostaglandins. The levels of linoleic acid, dihomo-gamma-linolenic acid (DGLA) and arachidonic acid are all deficient in the red blood cell membranes of schizophrenics. The delta-6-desaturase enzyme and the delta-5-desaturase enzyme both seem to be impaired as well, and this would interfere with the conversion of both linoleic acid into GLA, and of DGLA to prostaglandin E1. Instead, the arachidonic acid may be being used up to form series 2 prostaglandins at double the rate. This suggests that evening primrose oil may be able to help, because it bypasses the delta-6-desaturase enzyme by providing the body with GLA directly.

Dr Horrobin, who has done much of the British research into prostaglandins and evening primrose oil, first suggested that a deficiency of prostaglandin E1 may play an important role in the production of the symptoms of schizophrenia. There has been much clinical evidence to support this link and some of the discoveries made are summarised below:

* Schizophrenics get better when they develop fever or have seizures and both these states are associated with a rise in prostaglandin levels in the brain.

* Rheumatoid arthritis (which involves a rise in synovial or lubricating prostaglandins) and schizophrenia, are mutually exclusive diseases.

* Platelets taken from schizophrenics fail to turn dihomo-gamma-linolenic (DGLA) acid into prostaglandin E1.

* Schizophrenics have low levels of linoleic acid and DGLA, but have high levels of arachidonic acid which suggests that they convert dietary linoleic acid rapidly into arachidonic acid.

* A recent World Health Organization study carried out in eight centres showed that schizophrenia was less severe in countries where there was a higher proportion of unsaturated fat from fish, vegetables and seafood in the diet.

Sixty percent of patients on neuroleptic drugs suffer from motor disorder side-effects such as tardive dyskinesia. The involuntary movements can be extremely disabling. In a preliminary study carried out by Dr Vaddadi, it was observed that there was a sudden reduction in these involuntary movements in some of his schizophrenic patients while they were being treated with evening primrose oil and penicillin.

During open trials with EFAs, Dr Horrobin noticed that abnormal involuntary movements in some schizophrenics reduced or even disappeared. These and other clinical observations prompted Dr Horrobin to carry out a double-blind, placebo-controlled trial of Efamol evening primrose oil on a group of psychiatric patients, mainly chronic schizophrenics with abnormal involuntary movements. The study involved forty-eight patients, thirty-nine of whom were schizophrenic, four were manic-depressive and three had personality disorders. All of these patients had well-established movement disorders of at least mild severity. The patients had been given neuroleptic drugs for a minimum period of three months. This medication was kept constant except in five patients, three of whom were given a placebo, while two were given evening primrose oil. Thirty-eight patients completed the trial.

Blood was also taken from twenty age-matched non-psychiatric hospital controls and seventeen diagnostically matched psychiatric controls, none of whom suffered from involuntary movements. After a period of four weeks, the patients were randomly allocated to receive either a placebo or evening primrose oil for a period of sixteen weeks. Patients were given twelve capsules of Efamol daily. At the end of this period there was a crossover to the other treatment for a further period of sixteen weeks. The results showed that patients who had severe involuntary movements had the lowest values of omega-3 essential fatty acids (group of EFAs found in fish oil) and omega-6 essential fatty acids (group of EFAs found in vegetable oils including evening primrose oil); 81 percent of these psychiatric patients were schizophrenic.

The trial also revealed that schizophrenics who were given evening primrose oil had increased levels of dihomo-gamma-linolenic acid and arachidonic acid. No other individual fatty acids showed any significant change. At the end of the sixteen-week period all the patients were switched to receive evening primrose oil and Efavit tablets (containing ascorbic acid, pyridoxine hydrochloride, nicotinic acid and zinc sulphate). These micronutrients are known co-factors in the metabolism of EFA to prostaglandin E1. The combination of Efamol and Efavit produced more significant improvements than either placebo or evening primrose oil alone, in both mental state and abnormal movements. The memory of the patients taking this combined treatment improved and there was a significant rise in the levels of both omega-3 and omega-6 essential fatty acids. The Efamol capsules contained added vitamin E as well as evening primrose oil, which increased its effect on tardive dyskinesia (involuntary abnormal movements). It has been suggested that neuroleptic drugs can generate free radicals which destroy essential fatty acids, and vitamin E is a powerful antioxidant which restricts the formation of free radicals.

Diet

As with most other medical conditions, the diet of schizophrenics affects their symptoms. Cutting out wheat, milk and foods containing arachidonic acid, such as meat, dairy products and peanuts, has been of benefit to some patients. There are other nutritional factors also to be considered. Some doctors think that schizophrenics respond well to therapy with zinc and vitamin B6, in which they are often deficient. These nutrients can do little to help control behaviour or hallucinations, but can be effective in treating the lack of emotional contact in schizophrenics.

The link with epilepsy

Despite being under close medical scrutiny for many years, no serious side-effects have been linked with taking evening primrose oil. The most common complaint is a mild stomach upset and this can be relieved by taking the capsules with food. Some patients also report looser bowel movements as a result of taking the oil, which is probably not a bad thing. However, there is a small but persistent claim that crops up in the popular press linking evening primrose oil with epilepsy. So is there any truth in this story that threatens to undermine its medical credentials? The link with epilepsy stems from medical trials carried out several years ago. Over 300 people took part and three developed epilepsy during the trial. One patient was subsequently found to have been taking the placebo or dummy pill, so evening primrose oil could not have been the cause. The other two had been misdiagnosed as schizophrenics, when they were in fact suffering from epilepsy. However, because these cases came to light after the clinical trials they were mistakenly linked to evening primrose oil. Since then, epileptics who are prescribed evening primrose oil are monitored by their doctors as a precautionary measure, but no adverse reactions have been reported to date.

—9—
Evening Primrose Oil and Cancer

Evening primrose oil has even been shown to be helpful in cases of cancer, a disease which dominates many people's lives and which kills millions. Recent studies have demonstrated that evening primrose oil can selectively kill cancer cells without affecting normal cells. The traditional treatment for cancer, which involves radiation, kills both cancer cells and normal cells because it can not distinguish between the two types of cell. This treatment can also have chronic side-effects including total hair loss. Most of the studies carried out on evening primrose oil have taken place on animal and human cancerous cells in laboratories but there have been some trials on human cancer patients. Cancer patients are shown to have low levels of essential fatty acids in their blood and the delta-6-desaturase enzyme, which converts dietary linoleic acid into GLA, is blocked. When GLA is administered directly to the body, the level of essential fatty acids increases, and cancer cells are killed.

Lipid Peroxidation

Polyunsaturated lipids (fats) are highly susceptible to a process called lipid peroxidation. This process is like a chain reaction which can produce a whole series of highly reactive substances and a whole range of peroxidised lipids. This process of lipid peroxidation is widely regarded as harmful and is thought to play a role in cancer, rheumatoid arthritis and other inflammatory disorders, alcoholic liver damage, and many other conditions. However, if this process really is bad then administering highly unsaturated fatty acids should, in theory, make things worse by increasing the formation of the presumably damaging end products.

There has, though, been extensive evidence that contradicts this theory. As we have seen in this *Quick Guide*, countless clinical trials have revealed that administering essential fatty acids such as GLA, which bypass the delta-6-desaturase step, in inflammatory conditions and other disorders has demonstrated consistent improvements rather than deteriorations in the clinical state. This evidence seems to suggest that lipid peroxidation is not such a bad process after all. Many of the agents which have anti-cancer cell actions are also able to initiate increased peroxidation of unsaturated lipids.

As soon as a cell has become cancerous, it resists the process of lipid peroxidation, possibly because these cells contain large amounts of antioxidants like vitamin E. Cancer cells have very low levels of the delta-6-desaturated essential fatty acids such as GLA, and the more rapidly the cancer grows, the greater is the lack of these essential fatty acids. Tests on fibroblasts (cells in connective tissue) which were taken from mice, revealed that the most malignant cells contain the most saturated fatty acids, while the least malignant cells are much less saturated. Whenever there is a lack of essential fatty acids, the cell always compensates by creating more oleic acid, and therefore becomes even more saturated.

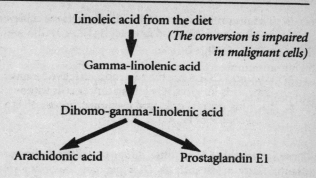

Linoleic acid from the diet

(The conversion is impaired in malignant cells)

Gamma-linolenic acid

Dihomo-gamma-linolenic acid

Arachidonic acid   Prostaglandin E1

Evening primrose oil and cancer

In the last ten years there have been experiments carried out by independent laboratories on over twenty human and some animal malignant cell lines, which are compared with about ten normal human and animal cell lines. The results have been consistent and are summarised below:

* When gamma-linolenic acid (GLA) is added to malignant cell lines, the cells die within four to ten days.

* This effect is time-dependent – the cultures need to be prolonged for more than twenty-four hours.

* Normal cells are not damaged.

* When normal cells are out together with human cancerous cells, the latter completely outgrow the former within ten days. When GLA is added, the reverse happens, with the malignant cells dying and being overwhelmed by the normal cells.

* The maximum cancer cell-killing effects are achieved by all natural omega-6 fatty acids (GLA, DGLA and AA – arachidonic acid).

* GLA and DGLA are the two most effective essential fatty acids in selectively killing cancer cells without harming normal cells, and evening primrose oil is a good source of GLA.

These experiments leave little doubt that delta-6-desaturated essential fatty acids such as GLA play an important role in combating malignant cells. All the studies carried out in laboratories revealed that by simply adding GLA to cells, the cancerous cells were killed off, while the normal cells did not suffer from the extra levels of GLA. These experiments were carried out in vitro, which means that cells were studied in a laboratory and not actually in a human. Although the results of these experiments are interesting and very encouraging, they do not offer proof that essential fatty acids will have the same effect in killing cancer cells in humans. As yet there have been a limited number of trials carried out in vivo (in humans) on the use of GLA, but these have been encouraging. It is difficult to give 6g of GLA per day in the form of evening primrose oil as this would require the administration of more than a hundred capsules. However, open studies have revealed that doses of up to thirty capsules of Efamol per day have been helpful. Much more research must be carried out to determine the most effective forms of essential fatty acids in conquering each type of cancer, and the most effective doses. However, it now seems that essential fatty acids could hold one of the clues in our quest for a safe cancer therapy in humans.

—10—

Evening Primrose Oil and Raynaud's Syndrome

This little-known condition causes a painful, tingling sensation in the fingers and thumbs. In severe cases, the hands and feet become abnormally cold and symptoms of a disease affecting the circulation such as atherosclerosis, or the connective tissue such as scleroderma, may occur. No one knows exactly what causes Raynaud's syndrome. The arteries contract in spasm which makes the fingers go pale and numb. This condition can become considerably dangerous as a lack of blood in the extremities can cause gangrene, or ulceration of the finger tips. Evening primrose oil can again come to the rescue with this strange condition. A study carried out at the Centre for Rheumatic Diseases at Glasgow Royal Infirmary revealed that six out of eleven patients found a definite benefit from evening primrose oil, while two patients felt a moderate benefit and three felt no benefit. The patients were given twelve capsules daily while ten other patients were given a placebo. As the weather deteriorated, the group taking the placebo experienced significantly more attacks than the patients who were taking the evening primrose oil.

Raynaud's syndrome is sometimes the first sign of scleroderma which is a rare disease affecting the body's connective tissue which supports and protects the organs of the body. Scleroderma causes the connective tissue to grow harder and contract. No one knows why this happens, but it is thought to be an auto-immune disease, where the body attacks itself. The disease usually strikes people in their thirties and it is three times more likely to affect women than men. Scleroderma can attack any part of the body, even the heart, kidneys or lungs, and it can either stay in one place or spread throughout the whole body.

Patients who have Raynaud's syndrome and scleroderma have been found to be lacking in prostaglandin E1 which seems to be caused by a blockage in the process which converts essential fatty acids into prostaglandins. Evening primrose oil can correct this problem through bypassing some of the areas where the blockage can occur.

How Evening Primrose Can Help Treat Raynaud's Syndrome and Scleroderma

Again, evening primrose is effective in treating these diseases because it produces prostaglandin E1 in the body. This prostaglandin has been used in the past as an effective drug in severe Raynaud's syndrome, showing an increase in hand temperature for up to six weeks. However, because these drugs have to be administered intravenously at a hospital, a less inconvenient method was sought instead.

Evening primrose oil was to be this new method of treating the disease as it not only enables the body to make its own prostaglandin E1, but also helps to keep cell membranes fluid and flexible. This is an important function in a disease such as Raynaud's syndrome and, because unsaturated fatty acids, such as the GLA in evening primrose oil do not solidify in the cold, it has added benefits.

——11——

Evening Primrose Oil
and Hyperactivity
in Children

Hyperactivity is a real strain on parents who feel that they never get the chance to relax, while their child seems to have an inexhaustible supply of energy. It is important to watch what hyperactive children eat; 94 percent of hyperactive children can be helped through diet. One of the most famous diets designed especially for hyperactive children is called the Feingold diet. It was invented by an American doctor named Feingold and there have been other good diets created since which are based on his method of eating. Hyperactive children should avoid any artificial colourings, flavourings and preservatives as well as natural salicylates which are found in most fruit such as apples, oranges, grapes, strawberries, peaches and cherries. Dried fruits are also high in natural salicylates. These salicylates are known to block the conversion of prostaglandins and so hyperactive children may be deficient in prostaglandin E1, which influences behaviour. These low levels of prostaglandins may be set right by taking evening primrose oil.

Blood samples taken from hyperactive children have shown reduced levels of dihomo-gamma-linolenic acid (DGLA – which goes on to produce prostaglandin E1). Evening primrose oil is, as we have seen, an excellent source of GLA and this converts into DGLA. Controlled trials using Efamol evening primrose oil in treating hyperactive children have shown great improvement in young children who suffered from mood swings, sleep disorders, crying spells, and general misery for no particular reason. Most of the children who responded well had some evidence of atopy (infantile eczema or asthma) or a family history of mood disorder or solvent/drug abuse. In some of the cases there was improvement only in their symptoms of atopic disorders, but in others there was improvement in mood swings.

Case Histories

T.K.

This nine-year-old boy was put on the trial because of hyperactivity, oppositional behaviour and specific reading difficulty. His mother suffered from a mood disorder. T.K. showed considerable variety in mood and would be moderately depressed for two or three weeks and then become hyperactive, overtalkative, and disinhibited. He said that he felt better when taking the evening primrose oil capsules and he continued to take them without parental supervision, so they must have been effective; he would even remind his mother when to get a new supply. His school reported that his concentration improved, as did his work.

R.M.

This ten-month-old baby was put on the trial because he screamed virtually all day and night, and the mother could no longer cope. She gave her baby into the hands of foster parents for fear that she might be driven to hurt her own child. The foster mother had considerable experience and she claimed that this child was the most difficult child she had ever fostered. On examination of the child, no abnormalities were apparent apart from the fact that he looked miserable, cried most of the time and would not participate in playful activities. Both of the maternal grandparents and four of the mother's siblings had histories of substance/ alcohol abuse. R.M. was given 250mg of Efamol evening primrose oil which was put on his cereal. After just forty-eight hours both the mother and health visitor telephoned separately to report that there had been a dramatic change in the child's behaviour. He became a normal, happy baby who smiled and enjoyed playing with toys. After one month the mother stopped giving him the evening primrose oil but she resumed the treatment after forty-eight hours as his screaming and misery had returned.

Treating children like these was not difficult as most children report that they feel better taking the supplements. Most of the younger children are unaware that they are taking it, because the oil can be spread on butter or margarine on bread and disguised by some other spread.

──12──

Conclusion

It is rare to find something such as evening primrose oil which can treat children and adults alike, no matter what age, for such a huge variety of different disorders, and without causing any harmful side-effects. The research continues into the benefits of this marvellous little flower, and who knows what future trials will reveal about its amazing effects? It is clear that evening primrose oil can make a real difference to many people's lives.

Glossary

AIDS – auto-immune deficiency is a disease in which the anti-bodies in the immune system treat cells in the body as foreign matter and destroy them.

Antioxidant – a substance that prevents oxidation. Nutrients with antioxidant activity include vitamin E, beta-carotene and vitamin C.

Arthritis – inflammation of one or more joints in the body causing painful swelling.

Atopy – a form of allergy such as eczema or asthma.

Cancer – any malignant tumour which arises from the abnormal and uncontrolled division of cells that invade and destroy the surrounding tissues.

Diabetes – a disorder where the body is unable to turn sugar into energy because of a lack of insulin.

Double blind – neither the patients in a clinical trial nor the doctors judging the results know what treatment each patient has been given.

Eczema – an inflammation of the skin which causes itching and red rashes.

Enzyme – a substance produced by the body that regulates biochemical reactions.

Essential fatty acid – unsaturated fatty acids which have eighteen, twenty or twenty-two carbon atoms in their chains and three, four or five double bonds. They can be converted within the body into larger and more highly unsaturated fatty acids which have important functions in the brain cells and other areas of the body. Some essential fatty acids are converted by the body into prostaglandins.

Free radical – a reactive particle that contains one or more unpaired electrons, causing it to be highly unstable and sometimes destructive within the body.

In vitro – when a study is carried out in a test tube in a laboratory and not carried out on humans.

In vivo – when a study is carried out on humans.

Lipid – a technical name for any type of fat, oil or other fatty substance.

Malignant – something which invades and destroys body tissue causing progressive deterioration and eventually death.

Metabolism – the sum of all the chemical and physical changes that take place within the body.

Multiple sclerosis – a chronic disease of the nervous system resulting in involuntary shaky movements of the limbs.

Oestrogen – a steroid hormone which controls female sexual development.

Oxidation – the process of using oxygen to release energy from cells. Its side-effect is to produce free radicals.

Phospholipids – a lipid (fat) containing a phosphate group as part of its molecule. Phospholipids are part of all tissues and organs, especially the brain, and they are involved in many of the body's metabolic processes.

Placebo – a dummy drug which will have no physical effect on patients. It is given to some patients in clinical trials so that the results of their treatment can be contrasted with the results of the patients taking the active drug.

Plasma – the straw-coloured fluid in which the blood cells are suspended.

Platelet – a disk-shaped structure present in the blood which has many functions including stopping any bleeding.

Polyunsaturates – fatty acids that contain several double bonds between carbon atoms in their chains.

Progesterone – a steroid hormone which is responsible for preparing the inner lining of the womb for pregnancy.

Prostaglandins – short-lived, hormone-like chemicals which regulate the activities of cells in the body.

Raynaud's syndrome – a condition in which the arteries of the fingers become cold and numb and enter spasm.

Schizophrenia – a severe mental disorder characterised by a disintegration of the process of thinking.

Thrombosis – a condition in which the blood changes from a liquid into a solid and forms a blood clot.

Trans-fats – fatty acids that have hydrogen and carbon atoms in a double bond on the opposite sides of their normal chains.

Useful Addresses

HEALTH SUPPORT GROUPS

Hyperactive Children's Support Group (HACSG),
71 Whyke Lane, Chichester, West Sussex PO19 2LD.
Tel: (01903) 725182

Multiple Sclerosis Therapy Centres, Unit 4, Murdock Road,
Bedford MK41 7PD. Tel: (01234) 325781

National Eczema Society, 4 Tavistock Place, London
WC1H 9RA. Tel: (0171) 388 4097

The Pre-Menstrual Tension Advisory Service, PO Box 268,
Lewes, East Sussex BN7 2QN. Tel: (01273) 487366

The Schizophrenia Association of Great Britain, Bryn Hyfryd,
The Crescent, Bangor, Gwynedd LL57 2AG.
Tel: (01248) 354048

Women's Nutritional Advisory Service, PO Box 268, Lewes,
East Sussex BN7 2QN. Tel: (0273) 487366

EVENING PRIMROSE OIL SUPPLIERS

Efamol, Efamol Marine and Efavit, manufactured by
Efamol Ltd, Efamol House, Woodridge House,
Woodridge Meadows, Guildford, Surrey. Tel: (01483) 578060

Distributed by Britannia Health Products Ltd, Forum House, 41–75 Brighton Road, Redhill, Surrey RH1 6YS. Tel: (01737) 773741

Naudicelle, manufactured and distributed by Bio-Oil Research Ltd, The Hawthorns, 64 Welsh Row, Nantwich, Cheshire CW5 5EU. Tel: (01270) 629323

Seven Seas, Hedon Road, Marfleet, Kingston Upon Hull, Humberside HU9 5NJ. Tel: (01482) 75234

To contact the Evening Primrose Office, tel: (0181) 740 1506

HERBAL OIL SUPPLIERS

The following supply calendula oil and St John's wort oil:

Neal's Yard Remedies; for mail order tel: (01865) 245436

Fleur Aromatherapy; for mail order tel: (0181) 444 7424

Index

HOW TO ORDER YOUR BOXTREE BOOKS BY LIZ EARLE

LIZ EARLE'S QUICK GUIDES
Available Now

☐	1 85283 542 7 Aromatherapy	£3.99
☐	1 85283 544 3 Baby and Toddler Foods	£3.99
☐	1 85283 543 5 Food Facts	£3.99
☐	1 85283 546 X Vegetarian Cookery	£3.99
☐	1 85283 989 9 Vitamins and Minerals	£3.99
☐	0 7522 1614 7 Herbs for Health	£3.99
☐	1 85283 984 8 Successful Slimming	£3.99

ACE PLAN TITLES

☐	1 85283 518 4 Liz Earle's ACE Plan The guide to antioxidant vitamins A,C and E	£4.99
☐	1 85283 554 0 Liz Earle's ACE Plan Weight-loss for Life	£4.99

All these books are available at your local bookshop or can be ordered direct from the publisher. Just tick the titles you want and fill in the form below.

Prices and availability subject to change without notice.

Boxtree Cash Sales, PO Box 11, Falmouth, Cornwall, TR10 9EN

Please send cheque or postal order for the value of the book, and add the following for postage and packing:

UK including BFPO – £1.00 for one book, plus 50p for the second book, and 30p for each additional book ordered up to a £3.00 maximum.

OVERSEAS including Eire – £2.00 for the first book, plus £1.00 for the second book, and 50p for each additional book ordered.

OR please debit this amount from my ACCESS/VISA Card (delete as appropriate).

Card number ☐☐☐☐☐☐☐☐☐☐☐☐☐☐☐☐

AMOUNT £ ....
EXPIRY DATE...
SIGNED ....
NAME ....
ADDRESS ....
....